What to Ask the Doc

The Questions to Ask to Get the Answers You Need

by
Margaret Fitzpatrick, RN, Linda Burke, RN, Daryl Lee, RN

ISBN: 0-9747002-0-7 (Paperback)

Library of Congress Control Number 2003092190

This book is printed on acid free paper.

Printed in the United States of America.

What to Ask the Doc

The Questions to Ask to Get the Answers You Need

by
Margaret Fitzpatrick, RN, Linda Burke, RN, Daryl Lee, RN

Table of Contents

Articles

Introduction

Countless sources of health-related information are available today: books, magazines, and the Internet all can be helpful resources. But specific information about your health should come from a healthcare professional who is familiar with you and your health history; it should come from your own doctor. *What to Ask the Doc*© gives you the essential tools for getting that information. It gives you knowledgeable questions—the kind of questions doctors and nurses ask when confronted with our own healthcare issues.

What to Ask the Doc© was written by critical-care nurses who recognized an urgent need for better communication between patients and healthcare providers. In our many years of nursing, we have seen that patients and their families are often overwhelmed by their healthcare experiences. As nurses, it is our goal to put patients and their families on a path to a more open dialogue with their healthcare providers.

The purpose of this book is not to give specific medical advice; that should come from your own doctor. Instead, by giving you the questions that we would ask, we can help you become an active partner in your healthcare experience. *What to Ask the Doc*© bridges the gap between patients and doctors by giving you *the questions to ask to get the answers you need.*™

How to Use This Tool

Part 1: Questions

The first section of this book provides lists of questions for over 70 different healthcare concerns. This is not an exhaustive treatment of every possible healthcare situation, but the questions can start a meaningful dialogue between you and your healthcare providers. While our book is called *What to Ask the Doc*© it is important to remember that many qualified healthcare professionals come together to provide care in hospital and outpatient settings. Nurses, respiratory therapists, dieticians, physical therapists, social workers, and other qualified professionals can help answer your questions.

Part 2: Articles

Part 2 of this book provides informative articles about selected healthcare topics. The articles are not intended to answer every question you might have, but they will give you a basic introduction to and understanding of a subject.

Getting the Information You Need

There are several ways to use this book:

Carry it with you to the doctor's office at your next appointment, or tear out or photocopy the pages you need to bring with you. Explain to the doctor that you have brought questions with you and that you would appreciate it if he or she would take some time to answer them.

Highlight the questions most important to you. You may not get the opportunity to ask all of the questions provided, so take a moment to pick the three or four that will give you the information you need most.

Write notes on the blank spaces provided when talking to your doctor—do not trust your memory. Often patients and family members think that they will remember complicated medical explanations and later regret not having taken the time to jot down a few notes.

Based on our experience as nurses, we believe that whatever the state of your health, you can benefit from better communication with your doctor. The questions are designed to help you open a more productive conversation with your doctor. You can look for answers to them in the written materials given to you by doctors and nurses, too. This book gives *the questions to ask to get the answers you need.*™ Make *What to Ask the Doc*© your companion on your healthcare journey.

What to Ask the Doc

The Questions to Ask to Get the Answers You Need

Acne Questions

What causes acne?

Should I see a dermatologist (a medical doctor who specializes in skin problems)?

What can I do to limit the amount of breakouts that I have?

Is acne caused by stress?

Can acne be made worse by allergies?

Are there foods that I should avoid?

Do you recommend that I take certain vitamins or supplements?

Do the over-the-counter creams help acne?

Is there prescription medication that can help my acne?

What are the advantages and disadvantages of taking this medication?

Should I avoid being in the sun?

Does having acne mean that my skin is not clean?

Should I wash with soap?

What makeup can I wear?

Should I use a moisturizer on areas of dry skin?

How can I avoid getting scars from the acne?

Where can I get more information about acne?

> **TIP** The American Academy of Dermatology has a web site with information at www.aad.org, as does WebMD on its web site at www.webmd.com. Just type in *acne* in the search box.

See also: Medication.

Attention Deficit/ Hyperactivity Disorder Questions

How is this condition diagnosed?

> **TIP** The American Academy of Pediatrics recommends collecting information about the child's symptoms in more than one setting (school, at home, and extracurricular activities are examples). It is also important to consider other diagnoses that may be causing problems similar to ADHD.

How many visits should we have (parent, child and doctor) before the ADHD diagnosis is made?

> **TIP** Recent guidelines from the American Academy of Pediatrics suggest three visits of at least 20 minutes each before a diagnosis is made.

Is medication always necessary to control the symptoms of ADHD?

What part does behavioral therapy play in treatment?

What changes do I need to make at home in order to help my child control his behavior and to focus better?

What changes should I make in my child's diet?

> **TIP** Although diet has not been shown to be a cure for ADHD it may be beneficial for you to consider the part that food additives, preservatives, and sweeteners play in your child's diet.

How should I involve the school, baby-sitter, day-care provider and school nurse in this treatment plan?

What side effects will this medication have on eating, sleeping and other routines?

Will this medication affect my child's physical growth?

How can I help my child cope with this diagnosis?

Will my child need to be on medication indefinitely?

How will we know when we can taper off the medication?

What does it mean if the medication is not working for my child?

Can that indicate that my child does not have ADHD?

Where can I look for more information about ADHD?

> **TIP** The American Academy of Pediatrics has a web site that has information about ADHD at www.aap.org, as does WebMD at www.webmd.com. Just type in *ADHD* in the search box.

See also: Medication.

Advance Directives/ End-of-Life Decisions

In the hospital, if your heart stops beating, your doctors and nurses are obligated to resuscitate you. The resuscitation method is called CPR (cardiopulmonary resuscitation/life support). If you have severe difficulty breathing the doctors will insert a breathing tube and connect it to a ventilator. Often ventilator support is called artificial respiration. In most circumstances this type of support is a temporary measure, which allows your body time to recover and heal.

There are circumstances that may occur where you are unlikely to recover from such events. Decisions need to be made regarding what type of support and what type of care you should receive.

An Advance Directive is a document that explains what type of support you want to receive if you are no longer able to communicate your wishes. There are several types of Advance Directives described below.

Types of Advance Directives

Living Will
A living will is a document that states what medical care and treatments you want and do not want if you are unable to speak for yourself. Every individual has the right to refuse or accept any medical care. The living will allows you to state if you want tube feedings, IV fluids, or medications to support your blood pressure. Living will forms can be found on the Internet, at your hospital, or from an attorney.

Do Not Resuscitate (DNR)
The attending physician writes a Do Not Resuscitate (DNR) order in the medical record. This order is written to let all healthcare

workers know that extraordinary measures are not wanted if the following events occur: a fatal arrhythmia, a cardiac arrest, or if your breathing stops. A DNR order can be written at any time when a patient, spouse or medical power of attorney, along with the doctor, decides that extraordinary measures are not wanted. Many hospitals have a policy that puts the DNR order on hold any time a person goes to surgery.

Healthcare Power of Attorney
Another way to be sure that your preferences are known in a medical emergency is to appoint a healthcare power of attorney (medical power of attorney or appointment of a healthcare agent). This individual is authorized to speak for you if you are unable to speak for yourself. In most states marriage automatically guarantees such status to a spouse. If you are not married or would like someone other than your spouse to make such decisions, you must legally assign this responsibility. Your preferences should be discussed with the person you select. Medical Power of Attorney forms can be obtained at your hospital, from an attorney or on the Internet.

Withdrawing of Support
Withdrawing of support is one of the most difficult situations that arise during hospitalization. The term *withdrawing of support* means to remove the ventilator, specific IV drugs and other medical interventions that sustain or prolong life. The decision to withdraw support is made when you are being kept alive with medical devices yet there is little or no hope for recovery to a desirable state of health. The decision to withdraw is made by your doctor and family (or medical power of attorney) and is only done with full understanding and consent.

Options for pain control should also be discussed when considering withdrawing support.

Having any type of Advance Directive helps your family to know your preferences. Oftentimes such conversations do not take place before hospitalization, leaving families to make difficult decisions without knowing the patient's intensions. Many people find that talking with the hospital chaplain, social worker or patient representative can provide instruction and support while making such difficult decisions.

These are decisions with legal implications. It is important to discuss this with your family and to write out your preferences. Be sure to have end-of-life-care documents witnessed and keep copies in a secure place where your family members can find them. It is important that these forms are brought with you and put into your chart any time that you are hospitalized.

In the United States many states host web sites that provide free information about Advance Directives. Search the web for information in your state. There are also web sites that, for a fee, provide forms that you can complete regarding end-of-life-care decisions. Be sure to consult a lawyer if you have legal questions.

More information can be found on the web site Hospice.net at www.hospice.net.

See also: Organ and Tissue Donation, Pain After Surgery or a Procedure, Getting Along in the Hospital, and Hospice Care.

Alzheimer's Disease Questions

How is this diagnosis made?

What tests need to be done to make a definitive diagnosis?

> **TIP** An absolutely definitive diagnosis cannot be made until an autopsy is done after death. There are tests that can be done, such as a CAT scan or an MRI, to rule out other diagnoses. You may want to ask for these tests to be sure that another problem is not being mistaken for Alzheimer's.

How is this different from dementia?

Is this a normal part of aging?

What causes this condition?

Is Alzheimer's always a fatal disease?

How quickly will this progress?

Is there anything that will slow the progression of this condition?

Should I see a neurologist (a medical doctor with advanced training in diseases of the brain and neurological system)?

Are there medications to help with the symptoms of Alzheimer's?

Are the medications a cure for the disease?

Should I change my diet?

Should I increase or decrease my level of activity?

Am I still all right to live independently?

What plans should my family and I be making for the immediate and long-term future?

What can I expect to happen over the next few months?

How often should I see the doctor?

Does Alzheimer's make me vulnerable to other illnesses?

> **TIP** It is common for Alzheimer's patients to suffer from depression. This can be quite severe. You may want to ask your doctor for a plan to help you and your family recognize and cope with depression.

Are my children more likely to get Alzheimer's?

What support groups are available to Alzheimer's patients and their families?

Is there a web site or book that I can read to learn more about Alzheimer's?

> **TIP** The Alzheimer's Foundation has a web site with information at www.alz.org.

See also: Medication, Depression, and Diagnostic Testing.

Anesthesia

Anesthesia is medication that is given to create a partial or complete loss of sensation or feeling. A licensed anesthesiologist or certified registered nurse anesthetist administers anesthesia. The following are types of anesthesia:

General

The patient is given medication so that he cannot feel anything and is unconscious.

General anesthesia usually requires an overnight hospital stay, the placement of a breathing tube and the assistance of a ventilator. Patients recovering from general anesthesia require monitoring and special nutrition. It is very common to be nauseated after general anesthesia; you should ask your anesthesiologist what medication you can receive to treat nausea.

You may not be allowed to eat or drink initially after surgery because general anesthesia causes a temporary decrease in normal bowel function. Your doctors and nurses will monitor your bowel sounds and determine what is best for you to eat.

Local

Medication given to prevent the feeling of painful sensation in a particular part of the body.

Many people have had a local anesthetic, such as Novocain, from a dentist.

Spinal

Anesthetic medication is given directly into the space around the spinal cord. This blocks pain sensations from below that point on the body.

Epidural

This is similar to a spinal anesthetic. Medication is injected into the space surrounding the spinal cord, temporarily blocking pain from below that point on the body.

The difference between spinal and epidural anesthesia has to do with the space where the medication is injected.

You will meet with your anesthesiologist before going to surgery. If possible, arrange to speak to your anesthesiologist several days before your procedure so you can have all your questions answered in advance. If it is impossible to meet with the anesthesiologist prior to the day of surgery, you can arrange to speak with him on the phone. It is important to share any information about your medical history, allergies and your alcohol intake. The anesthesiologist will have you sign a consent form for anesthesia after all your questions have been answered and you understand the process.

See also: Anesthesia Questions, Pain Questions and Advance Directives.

Anesthesia Questions

What are my options for the type of anesthesia?

What are the advantages and disadvantages of the type of anesthesia I will have?

How long will I be under anesthesia?

Where will I be when I wake up?

Will I have a breathing tube in place during surgery?

When will the breathing tube be removed?

What are the monitoring devices used to monitor me during surgery?

How will I feel when I wake up?

Will local anesthetic be used at the surgical site so that I will not have as much pain when I wake up?

TIP **This is a frequently used technique for orthopedic surgeries.**

What type of medicine will I be given for pain after surgery?

Can I expect to feel nauseated when I wake up?

Is there medication that I can be given before I wake up to prevent nausea?

Where will I go after surgery?

When is it safe for me to leave the hospital?

When is it safe for me to drive a car?

Can you recommend a web site or book that I can read for
more information?

> **TIP** The American Association of Nurse Anesthetists has an informative web site at
> www.anesthesiapatientsafety.com.

See also: Pain After Surgery or a Procedure, Pain Questions, Inpatient
Surgery, Outpatient Surgery and Advance Directives.

Arthritis Questions

What is arthritis?

How do you diagnose arthritis?

    TIP Frequently, a blood test, bone density scan, x-ray and/or MRI is ordered.

What type of arthritis do I have?

Does arthritis always get worse with time?

How is arthritis treated?

If medication is prescribed, will it cure the arthritis or is it used to control the symptoms?

Will this medication put me at risk for any other health problems?

Will I need an additional pain reliever?

Can I take additional ibuprofen and/or aspirin with the medication you have prescribed?

Are cold packs or heat therapy beneficial?

Will exercise help me with this condition?

Should I regularly attend physical therapy?

Will additional physical therapy help me during times of increased arthritis pain?

Will I need surgery in the future?

Should I lose weight to help ease the symptoms of arthritis?

What changes in my diet will help with my condition?

Will nutritional supplements help with the symptoms of arthritis?

Do you have any additional information for me to read about arthritis?

> **TIP** The Arthritis Foundation has a web site with more information at www.arthritis.org.

See also: Medication, Orthopedic Surgery, Diagnostic Testing, and Pain Questions.

Asthma Questions

What is asthma?

Will my child have asthma for the rest of his life?

Will medication be prescribed?

How do you decide when to prescribe oral medication?

What effect will these medications have on my child's health?

Will the medication affect my child's sleeping patterns?

Will the medication affect my child's appetite?

Should we keep an inhaler with us at all times (school, car, after-school activities)?

Is it best to use a spacer with the inhaler? Does that help children get a more exact dose of the medication?

> **TIP** Many asthma experts strongly suggest that children use a spacer to help with the inhaler.

What is a nebulizer? Should we have one at home?

If my child continues to have difficulty breathing after using the inhaler or nebulizer, what should we do?

How will I know that my child is having a severe asthma attack?

What are retractions?

When should I take my child to the emergency room?

What instructions should I give to my child's school?

When should my child be kept home from school?

What changes do I need to make at home to help control my child's asthma?

> **TIP** Many doctors recommend that children NOT be exposed to cigarette smoke. You may need to remove rugs that collect dust, and purchase new pillows that are allergen-free. Unfortunately, many children are allergic to family pets. In time, you will learn your child's asthma triggers.

What is peak flow testing and why is it important?

Is there any connection between diet and asthma?

Should my child be tested for allergies?

Do you have more information for me to read about asthma?

> **TIP** The American Lung Association has a web site with information at www.lungusa.org, as does the American Academy of Pediatrics, at www.aap.org.

See also: Asthma in Children, Medication, Pediatric Procedures/Testing, Emergency Room Visit Questions, and Emergency Room Article.

Asthma in Children

Asthma is one of the most common diseases in childhood and can be the leading cause of school absenteeism. It is important that children and the adults who care for them are well informed about what to do in the event of an asthma attack.

Asthma is characterized by a narrowing of the lower airway and difficulty breathing. The child may complain of a "tight" feeling in the chest, you may hear wheezing, or the child may have a severe cough. This can be caused by many things: allergies, fumes from paint or cleaning products, perfume, cigarette smoke, pets, colds—these are all referred to as asthma triggers. It is important for you and your child to be aware of what asthma triggers affect him.

Asthma can be a life-threatening condition. Most children with asthma live full and normal lives—although they may need to use an inhaler and/or take medication every day. It is very important that the adults in your child's life are aware of his asthma. Spend time with day-care providers, teachers and the school nurse, letting them know about your child's asthma triggers and treatment. Ask your doctor for a written asthma-management treatment plan to bring to school. It may be necessary for your child to keep an inhaler at school (check with your school regarding guidelines; some require inhalers to be kept in the office).

There are many resources available to help you and your child to learn about living with asthma. The American Lung Association has a web site with information at www.lungusa.org.

See also: Asthma and Medication.

Back Injury Questions

What is the nature of my injury?

How is this diagnosis made?

Do I need an MRI, CAT scan or x-ray?

How long will this injury take to heal?

Should I be using ice or heat therapy?

Do you recommend muscle relaxants?

What pain medication will be prescribed?

Should I limit the amount of Tylenol™ (acetaminophen) and ibuprofen that I take every day?

> **TIP** Exceeding the recommended dose of acetaminophen or ibuprofen can lead to liver or kidney damage. Discuss with your doctor or pharmacist all of the medications you are taking before starting a new prescription.

Will I require bed rest?

What is the best position (alignment) for sleep?

> **TIP** Some suggest that sleeping on the floor with legs elevated can provide comfort.

Do I need a back brace, and how long will I need to wear it?

When can I start sporting activities?

How much weight can I lift safely?

When can I start physical therapy, and what are the advantages and disadvantages?

Are there any alternative treatments for my back problem?

> **TIP** Some doctors recommend a chiropractor, acupuncture or herbal therapy.

Do you recommend that I lose weight to help my back?

How important is nutrition at this time in my life?

> **TIP** Be careful that the diet plan you follow allows a proper amount of protein, which is vital to healing and good cell formation.

Is it necessary to limit sexual activity for a period of time?

Will an airplane ride increase my back pain?

> **TIP** Swelling around the injured site may increase with pressure changes that occur in airplane travel.

Will a long car ride aggravate my back pain?

What exercises do you recommend to help strengthen my back and lessen pain?

> **TIP** Your doctor may recommend that you do the back exercises for the rest of your life.

Do you have any information that I can read about back pain?

> **TIP** The American Academy of Orthopaedic Surgeons has a web site with information at www.aaos.org, as does WebMD, at www.webmd.com. Just type in *back pain* in the search box.

See also: Pain After Surgery or a Procedure, Pain Questions, Diagnostic Testing, and Medication.

Broken Bone/Bone Fracture Questions

Where on the x-ray is the break in the bone?

What kind of break is it?

> **TIP** There are several different types of fractures: comminuted, greenstick, and spiral are examples. Ask your doctor to explain the type of fracture.

How will the fracture be reduced?

> **TIP** To reduce a broken bone means to bring the broken ends back into proper alignment.

Will this require surgery?

> **TIP** Open fractures (where the bone goes through the skin) will require surgery. Closed fractures that are complex may also require surgery.

What type of cast or method of immobilization (special wrapping or devices) will be used?

> **TIP** A broken bone must be kept from moving (immobilized) in order for the two ends of the bone to heal together properly.

Will I need traction?

Why is it important to keep the broken bone elevated?

What should I do if the area below the cast or wrapping has numbness, tingling or feels unusually cold?

What should I do if I get the cast wet?

How long will I need the cast?

Will I need to see a physical therapist after the cast is taken off?

Will I experience muscle spasms?

What can I do to relieve muscle spasms?

What should I do to relieve pain?

What should I do if I experience a sudden increase in pain?

Will I experience pain when the cast is removed?

Should I make changes in my diet to help the bone heal?

Will I receive a copy of the x-ray?

Do you have information for me to read about broken bones?

> **TIP** The American Academy of Orthopaedic Surgeons has a web site with information at www.aaos.org, as does WebMD, at www.webmd.com. Just type in the words *bone fracture* in the search box.

See also: Orthopedic Surgery, Pain After Surgery or a Procedure, Pain Questions, and Pediatric Procedures/Testing.

Cancer Questions

What are the recommended treatments for this type of cancer?

What are the alternative treatments that are available?

> **TIP** Some people benefit from other therapies such as massage, stress management, yoga and meditation.

What is the treatment that you would recommend for a member of your family?

Is it appropriate for me to enter a trial study of new treatments?

> **TIP** There are many trial programs for cancer patients wherein doctors give treatments that are under consideration for approval by the Food and Drug Administration. Your doctor may or may not recommend you for a trial program, depending on your circumstances and health profile. More information about trial studies can be found on the National Institutes for Health web site at www.nih.gov.

What percentages of people undergoing the recommended treatments live for more than five years after treatment?

What is the likely outcome if I do not seek treatment?

What lifestyle changes can I make that will improve my condition?

Are there changes in my nutrition that I should make?

> **TIP** Nutritional therapy for cancer is a controversial subject. However, there are few health conditions that do not benefit in some way by improving nutrition. This will not be a cure, but it can improve your overall health and allow your body additional strength in this time of stress.

Should other people in my family be screened for this type of cancer?

If surgery is recommended:

What postoperative complications do your patients most often experience after this surgery?

Am I vulnerable to complications?

> **TIP** Some patients are more likely to have complications. This can be true if you are obese, smoke cigarettes, drink alcohol excessively or have other medical problems.

What effect will the loss of the removed organ/tissue have on my entire body?

> **TIP** Removal of a part of your body will have consequences, and you will benefit from speaking to your doctor about this before surgery.

Can you give me the name(s) of patients that have undergone this surgery so I may talk with them about their experiences?

Are there support groups that I could go to and learn more about my condition?

Can you recommend a book or a web site where I can find more information?

> **TIP** The National Institutes of Health has a web site at www.nih.gov, as does the Centers for Disease Control and Prevention, at www.cdc.gov. WebMD may have information on its web site at www.webmd.com. Just type in the name of the cancer in the search box.

See also: Inpatient Surgery, Outpatient Surgery, Anesthesia, Medication, Pain After Surgery or a Procedure, Pain Questions and Advance Directives.

Cardiac Surgery Questions

Can you describe the surgery?

Who will be in the operating room?

> **TIP** Your surgeon usually works with a large team throughout your surgery.

Who will perform the surgery?

What are the risks involved in this surgery?

What are the most common complications?

Am I at risk for complications because of my health conditions?

> **TIP** Patients can be at greater risk for complications if they are obese, smoke cigarettes, drink alcohol excessively or have other health problems such as diabetes.

What is done to prevent complications?

What can I do before surgery to help prevent complications?

Should I make changes in my eating in the weeks before surgery?

> **TIP** Be sure to eat enough protein to help with healing and the formation of healthy cells and tissues.

Are there any alternatives to this procedure for me?

What will I have in or on my body when I wake up after surgery?

> **TIP** You may have a breathing tube, IV catheter, urine catheter, chest tube, staples or stitches, heart monitor, oxygen, nasogastric tube, pulse oximeter or surgical stockings.

When will these tubes come out?

Will I need to receive a blood transfusion?

If so, can I or my family members donate blood before my surgery?

TIP Blood donation from family must usually be done at least one week before surgery, and you will need your doctor's help to plan this step.

Should I take my regular medications, including aspirin, vitamins or insulin, the day of surgery?

What can I expect after surgery?

TIP In addition to all the various devices listed that may be required after surgery, you will probably be asked to do coughing and deep-breathing exercises every hour (while you are awake), walk in the halls with assistance, get up to a chair for meals, and you may have to take many new medications.

Can my visitors help me out of bed in the hospital? Can my visitors walk with me in the halls?

TIP When walking with a family member, ask your nurse what to do if dizziness occurs. Be sure to request pain medication 15 to 20 minutes before you get up if you feel discomfort. And ask how far you should walk.

How long will I be in the intensive care unit (ICU)?

Does the ICU have special visiting hours?

How long will I be in the hospital?

What happens when I am discharged?

What medication will I need to take after surgery?

How long will I need to take these medications?

What are the side effects for the medications that I am taking after surgery?

Will I be involved in a cardiac rehabilitation program?

Will a discharge planner or a social worker see me in the hospital?

Will anybody need to stay with me at home after I leave the hospital?

When can I start my normal activities (such as driving, exercise and sexual activity)?

Will I need to have special equipment at home?

Should I stop taking any supplements or medication that I am taking?

> **TIP** Aspirin, vitamin E, ibuprofen and Co-enzyme Q10 as well as other medications may prevent your blood from clotting properly (sometimes this is called thinning the blood). Ask your doctor about this if you take these medications.

Can you recommend a resource where I can get more information?

> **TIP** Johns Hopkins University Medical Center has information about cardiac surgery on its web site at www.csurg.som.jhmi.edu, as does the web site Heart Surgeon at www.heart-surgeon.com.

See also: Pain After Surgery or a Procedure, Pain Questions, Medication, Inpatient Surgery, Getting Along in the Hospital, and Discharge Planning.

Cerebral Vascular Accident (CVA or Stroke) Questions

What is a stroke?

> **TIP** There are different types of strokes. A stroke may be caused by a blood vessel breaking and leaking blood into the brain. Another type of stroke is caused by a blood clot that prevents oxygen from getting to a part of the brain.

What type of stroke did I have?

What makes me at risk to have a stroke?

What are the warning signs of a stroke?

> **TIP** If you experience unexpected weakness, especially on one side of your body, you should seek medical attention immediately. If you have a facial droop or difficulty seeing, walking or swallowing, you should contact your doctor, call 911 or have someone take you to the emergency room. It is important to seek medical attention as soon as possible to avoid serious complications.

What tests are done to diagnose a stroke?

> **TIP** Usually a CAT scan or MRI will be done to make a definitive diagnosis. You will also have blood tests in the hospital.

What medication is being given to prevent the stroke from getting worse?

> **TIP** If a clot in the brain causes the stroke, medication can be given to break up the clot; this is the case if treatment is given in the *first few hours* after the onset of symptoms.

Are anti-coagulants being given?

> **TIP** These are medications that are given to prevent abnormal clots from forming. They may be given to prevent a clot that can cause another stroke.

How is my heart rate and blood pressure being controlled? How will these vital signs be monitored while I am in the hospital?

What is an acceptable heart rate and blood pressure in these circumstances?

Why is it important to keep the heart rate and blood pressure from being too high or too low?

> **TIP** High blood pressure can put stress on the blood vessels in the brain; low blood pressure may prevent adequate flow of blood to the brain. An abnormal heart rate can also stress the body. Ask your doctor about these essential issues.

What part of my brain is affected by this stroke?

Can you show me how the stroke appears on a CAT scan? Can I get a copy of the CAT scan?

Can you give me a copy of the blood tests that have been done?

> **TIP** This is good to have in order to compare with other blood tests that you may have in the future and to show to doctors who may care for you in the future. Copies of blood test results are easily obtained by computer printout, and there is usually no delay to receive them while you are in the hospital. Getting results from outpatient tests is more time-consuming.

Is my life in danger because of this stroke?

Will I need surgery?

Will I require new medications because of this stroke?

What kind of rehabilitation will I need to recover from this stroke?

What deficits do I have from this stroke?

> **TIP** Deficits can include the loss of speech, continued weakness or the inability to use a limb.

What complications am I likely to have in the hospital? What is being done to avoid these complications?

How long will I be in the hospital?

What physical therapy will I receive in the hospital?

> **TIP** Physical therapy is very important for recovery from a stroke. Even very ill patients in the intensive care units can receive physical therapy. Patients who are unstable with very high or very low blood pressure may not be able to tolerate some forms of therapy, but it is an important part of care for most patients.

Will I be helped out of bed every day?

> **TIP** It is important to be getting out of bed frequently. This can help to prevent complications after a stroke. If you are in bed you may develop bedsores, lose more muscle tone, and it can even make you vulnerable to pneumonia. Even patients in the ICU are able to get into a chair unless their vital signs are unstable.

When will I work with a speech pathologist?

> **TIP** Speech therapy can be an important part of recovering from a stroke if it affects the speech centers of the brain. Speech pathologists can assist in helping stroke victims recover the ability to speak, learn alternative forms of communication and can also assist in the detection and treatment of problems with swallowing that can happen after a stroke. Speech therapy should begin as soon as the patient is able to participate, if there are not medical concerns that prevent it.

Will a dietician evaluate my nutrition in the hospital?

> **TIP** Adequate nutrition is vital to recovery. If you have problems swallowing or cannot eat on your own, you may need tube feedings. It is important that you have nutrition every day. Plain IV fluid is not nutrition; be sure to ask your doctor about how your nutritional needs are being met.

How will pain be assessed and treated?

> **TIP** After a stroke some patients have neurogenic pain, i.e., pain caused by damage to nerves. This requires special treatment, and you may need to ask to have a pain specialist treat you. Most hospitals have pain specialists.

After discharge from the hospital will I need to go to a rehabilitation facility or a nursing home? How is that decision made?

What services will I need when I get home from the hospital?

Is there someone at the hospital that can help me and my family prepare for my discharge?

Should I make changes in my diet to avoid another stroke?

> **TIP** If you are overweight, you are at a higher risk for the health problems that cause strokes.

Is there a support group that my family or I can attend to help us understand strokes and the adjustments that may be necessary?

Can you recommend a web site or book that I can read for more information?

> **TIP** The Stroke Association has a web site with information at www.strokeassociation.org, as does the Centers for Disease Control, at www.CDC.gov.

See also: Medication, Getting Along in the Hospital, Inpatient Surgery, and Diagnostic Testing.

Chronic Fatigue Syndrome (CFS) Questions

What causes CFS?

How is this diagnosis made?

> **TIP** Currently, there is not one definitive test for CFS. The diagnosis is usually made after ruling out other possible causes of symptoms.

Is there a physician that specializes in CFS that you can recommend?

How will you rule out mononucleosis, multiple sclerosis, lupus, depression, a systemic yeast infection, chronic sinusitis or another disease that may have similar symptoms?

What blood tests will be done?

Am I anemic?

> **TIP** This is determined by a blood test called a CBC (complete blood count).

Do I have an increased white blood cell (WBC) count?

> **TIP** This is also shown in a CBC. An increased white blood cell count can indicate infection.

Is my blood glucose level normal?

> **TIP** Blood glucose that is too high or too low can cause symptoms similar to CFS.

Should I have my hormone levels checked?

> **TIP** Hormone levels affect every aspect of well-being. Your doctor may recommend that you have additional blood tests to determine if your hormones are at the correct levels.

Should I make changes in my diet to increase my energy?

Do you recommend vitamins or other supplements?

What types of exercise or activity should I participate in?

Will you prescribe antidepressants? Can these increase fatigue?

Should I join a support group or get counseling?

How long does CFS last? When can I expect to return to my normal activities?

Do you have information that I can read about CFS?

> **TIP** The National Institutes of Health has a web site with information at www.niaid.nih.gov/factsheets/cfs.htm. There is also information on WebMD at www.webmd.com. Just type in *CFS* in the search box.

See also: Medication, Diagnostic Testing, and Depression.

Congestive Heart Failure (CHF) Questions

What is CHF?

What makes me vulnerable to CHF?

> **TIP** People who have had heart attacks are more likely to have congestive heart failure than are other people.

How is this diagnosis made?

Once I am diagnosed with CHF, will I always have it?

What are the signs/symptoms that I should call my doctor or go to the emergency room?

> **TIP** If you have swollen feet, difficulty breathing, or have to sit up to sleep, you need to contact your doctor. These are symptoms that you have extra fluid that can become a major problem if it is not corrected.

Why are my lungs and breathing affected by CHF?

How will the medications that I take help my CHF?

Which are the most important medications for my heart?

Will it hurt me if I do not take my medication for a few days?

Should I take vitamins or other health supplements?

How does my diet affect my CHF?

Should I speak to a dietician about the foods I eat?

Will exercise help my heart? What are the right kinds of activities for me to do to help my heart?

> **TIP** Almost every chronic health problem can be improved with the right types of exercise. Be sure to have your doctor's approval before you begin a new exercise/activity routine.

Does my weight affect my heart?

Is it important for me to weigh myself daily?

Is it important for me to keep track of how much I urinate?

Should I let the doctor know if I am not urinating as much as I am used to?

Where can I get more information about this condition?

> **TIP** There is more information on the Heart Failure web site at www.heartfailure.org, and on WebMD at www.webmd.com.

See also: Medication, Diagnostic Testing, Emergency Room Article, and Emergency Room Visit Questions.

Deep Vein Thrombosis (DVT or Blood Clot) Questions

A blood clot that forms in the deep veins that partially or completely blocks the flow of blood, most typically found in the calf or thigh.

What causes a DVT (blood clot)?

What makes me vulnerable to a DVT?

> **TIP** There are several risk factors for forming a blood clot, including: smoking, traveling in a car, train or airplane for an extended period of time, obesity and pregnancy.

Does having one DVT make it more likely that I will get another one in the future?

Why does having surgery increase the risk for getting a DVT?

What is done before and after surgery to prevent a DVT?

What tests are done to diagnose a DVT?

What blood tests will I have, and how will they help in the diagnosis?

Can you determine the size of the blood clot?

Why is this a dangerous condition?

How can we prevent the clot from moving to my lungs or other vital organs?

> **TIP** Ask your doctor about a Greenfield filter. This can be inserted in the large vein of the affected leg and can prevent the clot from traveling; it may or may not be an appropriate treatment for you.

Will I need a surgical procedure?

Will I receive medications to dissolve the clot?

How long will I be in the hospital?

What medications will I be taking when I get home?

Can I continue my current medications with the new one(s)?

Are there medications or vitamin supplements that I must avoid while taking this new medication?

How can I prevent getting another DVT?

Does my weight or eating habits make me vulnerable to another DVT?

What are the important danger signs that I must be aware of with this condition?

Do you have information for me to read about deep vein thrombosis, or a web site where I can obtain more information?

> **TIP** The Centers for Disease Control and Prevention has information on its web site at www.cdc.gov, as does WebMD, at www.webmd.com. Just type in *DVT* in the search box.

See also: Medication, Diagnostic Testing, and Getting Along in the Hospital.

Depression Questions

What are the causes of depression?

How can I tell if my depression is caused by a situation or by a chemical imbalance in my brain?

> **TIP** Situational depression can be the result of upsetting events, such as a death in the family or a divorce; chemical depression can be made worse during a time of life crisis, but it originates in the brain.

What symptoms of depression do I have?

> **TIP** There are several symptoms, such as difficulty sleeping or difficulty staying asleep, poor self-image, loss of appetite or excessive eating, decrease in sexual desire, suicidal thoughts, difficulty controlling emotions, lack of emotional feeling, and inability to enjoy activities that were once enjoyable. The symptoms for children are different; ask your pediatrician for help if you think your child may be depressed.

Can medication help me to recover from depression?

How do you decide what medication and what dose to prescribe?

How long will the medication take to work?

> **TIP** Many antidepressants can take 3 to 6 weeks to be effective.

What can I do to feel better while waiting for the medication to work?

Should medication be used together with talk therapy?

Can you recommend a therapist?

Is there an effective alternative to taking prescribed medication?

How will my family or I know if the depression is severe and possibly dangerous?

What should we do if the depression is becoming severe?

Are there other illnesses that may be causing my symptoms?

TIP There are hormonal imbalances that can cause depression-like symptoms.

Am I likely to have episodes of depression for the rest of my life?

Can changes in my diet help my depression?

How is my depression likely to affect my children?

What can I do to minimize the effect on my children?

Is it likely that my children will have depression now or as they grow older?

What are the signs of depression in children?

What support group would you recommend for me?

Where can I get more information about depression?

TIP The National Institute for Mental Health has information on its web site at www.nimh.nih.gov, as does WebMD, at www.webmd.com. Just type in the word *depression* in the search box.

See also: Medication.

Diabetes

The American Diabetes Association defines diabetes as a "disease in which the body does not produce or properly use insulin. Insulin is a hormone that is needed to convert sugar, starches and other food into the energy needed for daily life. The cause of diabetes is a mystery, although both genetics and environmental factors such as obesity and lack of exercise appear to play roles."

Diabetes is a condition in which your body cannot use food properly. When you eat, your body turns some of the food into glucose. Glucose enters the bloodstream and must team up with insulin to help the body use glucose for energy. Insulin helps the cells to accept glucose to be used for energy and also is the hormone responsible for fat storage.

Type 1 Diabetes:
The pancreas makes little or no insulin. People with Type 1 diabetes must take insulin daily for the rest of their lives.

Type 2 Diabetes:
The pancreas makes some insulin but not enough, or the body cannot properly use the insulin it makes—this is known as insulin resistance. This is the most common form of the disease.

It is important to know that keeping your blood sugar levels within a target range can prevent or delay the onset of many complications of the disease. Your doctor will tell you what that target range should be and how often you must check your blood sugar at home.

Complications caused by diabetes:
• Cardiovascular (the heart and the vessels outside the heart).
• Skin problems (problems with healing).
• Kidney disease, including kidney failure, which could lead to
  the need for dialysis or transplant surgery.
• Gum disease and infection.
• Nerve damage.
• High blood pressure.
• Foot problems and amputations due to infections.
• Eye disease and blindness.
• Stroke.
• Smoking cigarettes can increase the risk of
  developing complications.

There are 16 million people in the U.S. who have diabetes. Five million are not diagnosed, and many more have a condition referred to as pre-diabetes. More information can be found on the American Diabetes Association's web site at www.diabetes.org.

See also: Diabetes – Type 2, Medication, and High Blood Pressure.

Diabetes – Type 2 Questions

How is this diagnosis made?

What causes Type 2 Diabetes?

What is insulin resistance?

What part does my weight play in diabetes?

What should my blood sugar be?

> **TIP** Your doctor should give you information about what is a good blood sugar target range.

Why is it important that my blood sugar levels be in the target range?

> **TIP** High, uncontrolled blood sugar levels can kill you from the inside. It is vitally important to your long-term health that you control your blood sugar levels.

How will I monitor my blood sugar?

> **TIP** Blood sugar monitoring units can be bought at most pharmacies. Ask your doctor if you will need a prescription for the monitoring unit and supplies. Medicare and Medicaid, as well as other insurance, may help to pay for the cost of the supplies.

How often should I check my blood sugar?

> **TIP** Patients are more successful in controlling their blood sugar if they check it several times each day.

Should I keep a written diary of my daily blood sugar readings?

What should my family and I know about the warning signs of high blood sugar and low blood sugar?

> **TIP** High blood sugar (hyperglycemia) is a condition that causes damage over a period of time. People frequently feel very thirsty with high blood sugar and need to urinate often. Untreated, very high blood sugar can lead to coma. Low blood sugar (hypoglycemia) is a condition that can come on very quickly. You may feel tired, shaky, nervous or confused. This is a situation that needs fast action because it can be life-threatening. This is why it is important to be able to check your blood sugar. Ask your doctor for advice about how to handle these situations. Be sure that your family is aware of these important issues.

Should I attend a self-management class for diabetics?

> **TIP** These classes are offered in many communities; call your local hospital to ask if it hosts a meeting.

Is it important for me to change my eating habits?

Will you recommend a dietician for me to see?

> **TIP** You did not develop Type 2 Diabetes overnight, and it may not be easy for you to adjust your diet. Be sure to ask for as much help as you need to protect your health.

Will I be prescribed medication to help control my blood sugar?

What are the side effects of this medication?

Do the other medications that I am taking affect my body's ability to control blood sugar?

> **TIP** Some medications given to control high blood pressure and cholesterol may affect blood sugar levels; however, never stop taking any prescribed medication without consulting your physician.

How does exercise help to control my blood sugar? What type of exercise do you recommend for me?

How often should I see the doctor?

How will you monitor my diabetes?

What is a glycosylated hemoglobin test? How often will I have this done?

> **TIP** Your doctor must order this blood test. It measures how well your blood sugar has been controlled over the past two to three months.

What does a high glycosylated hemoglobin indicate?

Why do you test my urine?

Should I be testing my urine at home?

What other medical problems am I at risk for because of the diabetes?

What is peripheral neuropathy?

Do I need to take special care of my feet?

> **TIP** Because of diabetes, you may be at an increased risk for infections in your feet. Many doctors recommend that diabetic patients avoid wearing sandals or going barefooted, because even a small sliver may present a serious problem.

Will you recommend that I see a podiatrist (a doctor who specializes in care of the feet)?

Should I wear a medic-alert bracelet?

Where can I get more information about diabetes?

> **TIP** The American Diabetes Association has a web site with information at www.diabetes.org, as does the Centers for Disease Control and Prevention, at www.cdc.gov/diabetes. More information can be found on the WebMD web site at www.webmd.com. Most bookstores have many books on the subject in their health sections.

See also: Diabetes, Medication, Emergency Room Article, and Emergency Room Visit Questions.

Diagnostic Testing:
MRI, CAT Scan, X-ray Mammogram,
Biopsy or Lab Testing Questions

If you did not get your questions answered in the doctor's office, you may call and ask to speak with the doctor before you schedule the test.

Why is this test necessary?

What will you be looking for in the results?

Should I schedule this for a certain time of day?

Where do I call to schedule the tests?

> **TIP** When you call to schedule the tests, be sure to ask about parking information and ask for the specific information about where to go on the day of the test.

Can I eat and follow my usual routine prior to the test?

Should I bring someone with me for emotional support?

> **TIP** If you decide not to bring someone with you, be sure to have paper and pencil to write down any new information that the doctor may give you.

How long will the test take?

> **TIP** It is a good idea to bring a book or magazine with you to help pass the time.

Will I be enclosed in a machine for the test?

> **TIP** Some MRI machines are long tubes; others are open and do not fully enclose the patient.

Should I have sedation before the test if I feel anxious?

TIP You may feel nervous about the test; some physicians will prescribe a sedative to help you relax. If you take a sedative prior to the test, you will need to arrange for someone else to drive you to and from the test.

When will I know the results of the test?

Should I call the doctor's office to get the results, or will the office notify me?

TIP If you do not hear back from your doctor's office in the time specified, you might want to call to ask about the results.

Do you have any additional information that I can read about this type of test?

TIP The Radiological Society of North America has a web site with information about MRI, MRA, CAT scan, x-ray, mammogram and other radiology topics at www.radiologyinfo.org. WebMD also has information on its web site at www.webmd.com. Just type in the name of the test in the search box.

Discharge Planning Questions

Planning for discharge from the hospital can begin as soon as you are admitted. Hospitals have a number of ways to help you prepare to go home. It does not have to be stressful if your discharge is well planned. Many hospitals employ social workers, case managers and discharge planners to help prepare for the transition from hospital to home. Ask to be seen by one of them a few days before your scheduled discharge so that, when it is time to return to your home, you can do so with ease.

A family member can also request to meet with a discharge planner. It can be beneficial to do this almost immediately after the patient is admitted to the hospital or as soon as you know that the patient will be stable enough to be discharged. Many families have horror stories of receiving telephone calls stating that grandma was to be discharged the next morning and the family had to scramble to make arrangements. Think ahead and ask for help early so that this will not happen to you.

Medication:
Ask if you can receive the prescriptions prior to the day you leave so that a family member can pick them up before you arrive home. Another option is to ask to have your prescription phoned in to your pharmacy prior to your discharge. Many hospital pharmacies can prepare your prescription so that it is ready before you leave the hospital.

Follow-up Appointments:
Appointments with your physician can be scheduled before you leave the hospital, when it seems like there isn't much else to do but sit and wait. Ask which doctors you will need to see after you are discharged, request the office telephone numbers and make the appointments.

Lab work:
You may want to ask the following questions.

Will I need to have my blood drawn after I go home?

Where can I have this done closest to my home?

Do I need a doctor's order for this to be done?

How do I get my lab results?

Dieticians:
Dieticians play an important role in educating and preparing you for your discharge. You and/or your family member may ask to be seen by the dietician and request a written plan so that you know what foods are important to eat and what kinds of food must be avoided.

Visiting Nurse.
Some people discharged from the hospital have dressing changes or other medical treatments that must be continued at home by a registered nurse. Your doctor must write an order for these visits.

Be Sure to Ask:
How many visits will I have once I am discharged?

Does my insurance cover the cost of these visits?

Is my family expected to perform dressing changes or other medical procedures once I am discharged?

Who is responsible for teaching my family to perform the dressing changes?

Written Information:
Request that your doctors or nurses provide you with written

instructions when you are discharged. Your written instructions should include:

Medications:
What you are taking them for and what side effects to be aware of.

Follow-up Appointments:
With what doctors or therapist, and their telephone numbers so you can make the appointment.

Instructions:
Including information about dressing changes or other medical procedures that must be done at home.

Lab work:
Requires a doctor's written order; it should be written what the test is for and how often it is to be done.

Dietary Orders:
What special dietary restrictions you must follow.

Transportation Home:
If it is difficult for your family to transport you home, arrangements can be made for pickup by non-emergency ambulance. For some patients this is paid for by Medicaid/Medicare or other insurance, or you may have to pay the cost yourself. A discharge planner can help to answer these questions.

If possible, before you are discharged, have family or a friend take home plants, flowers, gifts and extra belongings. Be sure to have comfortable clothes to wear home. If you are taking pain medication, ask your nurse to give it to you just prior to leaving so that it is easier to move and get in and out of automobiles.

See also: Getting Along in the Hospital.

Ear Infection (Otitis Media) Questions

What causes an ear infection?

What are the symptoms of an ear infection?

Should I invest in an inexpensive home otoscope (instrument to examine the ear)?

Does giving my child a bottle in bed increase the risk of ear infection?

Does having cigarette smoke in the house increase my child's risk of ear infection?

How does swimming affect an ear infection?

What are adenoids?

Does this infection affect my child's adenoids?

How are ear infections treated?

Do you prescribe antibiotics for this condition?

How do we know if a virus or bacteria causes the ear infection?

TIP Antibiotics are only effective in treating infections caused by bacteria.

What are the risks associated with using antibiotics when they are not necessary?

What should I give my child to relieve the pain associated with ear infections?

How can I prevent ear infections?

> **TIP** Good hand-washing practices for you and your child will help to reduce the spread of infections.

Will giving my child an antihistamine or decongestant at the first signs of a cold help to avoid an ear infection?

Do you recommend that my child take a multivitamin every day?

How many hours of sleep should my child be getting each night?

Do you have information that I can read about ear infections?

> **TIP** The American Academy of Pediatrics web site has information at www.aap.org, as does the WebMD web site, at www.webmd.com.

See also: Medication, Fever in Children, Emergency Room Article, and Emergency Room Visit Questions.

Emergency Room

The first healthcare professional you will deal with will most
likely be the triage nurse. Usually a registered nurse, the triage
nurse will be the person who will take your vital signs and listen to your
description of your health problem. It is extremely important that you:

Have a complete list of your current medications, including any vitamin
or herbal supplements that you take. It is not necessary to bring the
bottles of medication, but always keep a current list of your medication
names and the doses with you.

Tell the triage nurse your complete medical history, including past
surgeries and hospitalizations.

Give a complete description of the symptoms that brought you to the
ER, when they started, and how severe they have been.

Tell the nurse if you are in pain, and rate that pain on a 0 to 10 scale: 0
is no pain and 10 is the worst you can imagine.

In the emergency room there is usually a wait to see a doctor. Patients
are not taken in to see the doctor based on when they came in, but
rather, based on the seriousness of their condition. You may see someone
who looks fine being taken in before you—but that person may have a
serious condition or medical history that needs immediate attention.

Do not eat or drink while you are waiting to see the doctor unless the
triage nurse gives you the okay. Ask the triage nurse if you will need to
provide a urine sample. If you have pain in your abdomen, urinary
problems or may be pregnant, they will probably need a urine specimen.

It can be especially important not to give children who may have a broken bone anything to eat or drink. They may need anesthesia to get the bone set, and if they have a full stomach this could cause serious complications. This is true for adults who may need anesthesia also.

The emergency room is a very busy place. It is best to not have a lot of people with you. If you have children who do not need to be seen in the ER, it is better for them to be at home with a responsible adult. If you do have several family members with you, please be aware that they will be asked to wait in the waiting room. Usually, you will be allowed one person with you. This is to be sure that the hallways are clear in the case of a medical emergency.

See also: Emergency Room Visit Questions, Pain After Surgery or a Procedure, Pain Questions, Medication, and Getting Along in the Hospital.

Emergency Room Visit Questions

There are many circumstances that may bring you to the emergency room. For more information, please refer to the Emergency Room Article.

The following questions are appropriate for most occasions for children and adults.

For the Triage Nurse:

> **TIP** The triage nurse is usually the first healthcare professional you will speak to in the ER.

How long will it be before I am able to see a doctor?

May I eat or drink while I am waiting to see the doctor?

Who should I go to if my symptoms become much worse while I am waiting?

Will the doctor need a urine specimen? Where can I give one?

If you feel that you need these things while waiting, ask the triage nurse for:
• a wheelchair
• an ice pack
• a container in case you vomit

For the Doctor or Nurse Treating You:

What tests will be ordered for me? Examples are: EKG, CAT scan, x-rays, and MRI.

Will I need blood tests?

What information will the tests give you?

Will I need an IV? Can the blood tests be drawn at the same time the IV is started so that I only need one needle stick?

How long do you expect this process to take?

Do you think that I will be admitted to the hospital?

Will you be speaking with my primary doctor?

How can I prevent coming to the emergency room in the future?

If you want more information about visiting the emergency room, go to the American College of Emergency Physicians web site at www.acep.org. WebMD also has information on its web site at www.webmd.com.

See also: Emergency Room Article, Pain Questions, Diagnostic Testing, Medication, and Inpatient Surgery.

Emphysema/Chronic Obstructive Pulmonary Disease (COPD) Questions

According to the American Lung Association, there are 1.8 million people in the United States with emphysema. There are over 17,500 deaths in the U.S. each year from this serious disease.

What are the causes of emphysema?

How is this diagnosis made?

What changes are happening in my lungs with emphysema?

Does this condition always get worse over time?

What changes in my health can I expect over the next few months?

Does this condition make me susceptible to other health problems?

Is there medication that I can take to help me to feel better?

> **TIP** If your doctor prescribes an inhaler, ask if you may use a spacer; it is recommended for use with inhalers to deliver an accurate dose of the medication.

How can I prevent or slow the progression of emphysema?

> **TIP** Most commonly, people with emphysema either are current or former smokers. If you smoke, it is VERY important that you stop immediately. Emphysema is a condition that can seriously impact your health.

Should I start an exercise program to help me with my breathing and overall conditioning? Is there a professional I should consult to help me with a program?

Does my weight and nutritional status affect my emphysema?

Will I need to be on supplemental oxygen at home?

What is my oxygen saturation level (pulse oximeter reading)?

> **TIP** Most people with emphysema will have a lower-than-normal oxygen saturation reading. It is important to know what your particular level is so that if you go to the hospital you can let the doctors and nurses know what is normal for you.

What would indicate that I need to go to the emergency room?

Is there information that I can read to learn more about emphysema?

> **TIP** The American Lung Association has an informative web site at www.lungusa.org.

See also: Medication, Diagnostic Testing, Emergency Room Visit Questions, and Emergency Room Article.

Fever in Children Questions

How should I take my child's temperature?

What is considered a fever?

What should I give my child when she has a fever?

Should I ever NOT treat a fever?

Do you recommend cool baths to reduce a fever?

At what point is a fever dangerous?

What are the signs of dehydration?

How much should my child be drinking to avoid dehydration?

What are the best liquids for my child to drink?

Is it important that my child eat solid food when she has a fever?

What should I be prepared to do if my child has a febrile seizure?

Should I call the doctor or go to the emergency room if my child develops a rash with the fever?

Should I dress my child in very warm clothing when there is a fever?

Do you have any other information I should read about fevers in children?

TIP The American Academy of Pediatrics has a web site with more information at www.aap.org, as does WebMD, at www.webmd.com.

See also: Medication, Emergency Room Visit Questions, and Emergency Room Article.

Fibromyalgia Questions

A chronic pain syndrome of unknown cause; patients typically have sore joints, irritable bowel syndrome, fatigue, difficulty sleeping and depression.

Who is most likely to develop this condition?

How is the diagnosis made?

> **TIP** Some specialists use the presence of tender points to diagnose fibromyalgia. If a patient consistently has 11 hypersensitive tender points, then a positive diagnosis can be made.

Could this be another condition that is mistaken for fibromyalgia?

Should I see a specialist to help me with this condition?

What role does stress play in this condition?

Does fibromyalgia get worse over time?

Will I have periods of remission (when the disease and the symptoms are not as noticeable)?

Does having fibromyalgia make me vulnerable to developing other serious health problems?

What treatments are recommended?

> **TIP** Frequently, patients improve with the use of low-dose antidepressants and non-steroidal anti-inflammatory drugs (such as ibuprofen).

Is it important to combine psychological counseling with the medical treatment?

How can I help my family and employer understand this condition?

Should I make changes in my diet to improve my health?

What sort of exercise program can help with the symptoms of fibromyalgia?

Are there support groups, web sites or other sources of information that you can recommend?

> **TIP** The Fibromyalgia Network has information on its web site at www.fmnetnews.com, as does WebMD, at www.WebMD.com. Type in *fibromyalgia* in the search box.

See also: Medication, Diagnostic Testing, and Depression.

Gall Bladder Disease Questions

What functions does the gall bladder perform?

What is the cause of my gall bladder disease?

Is there anything I can do to reduce the symptoms I am experiencing?

What can I do to relieve the pain I feel?

What foods should I be eating?

What foods should I avoid?

Will losing weight reduce the risk of reoccurring symptoms?

Does exercise reduce the severity of symptoms?

Is surgery recommended?

What are the treatment options for this disease other than surgery?

Will I be taking new medications for this condition?

Do you recommend any books or web sites that can help me learn more about this disease?

> **TIP** The Centers for Disease Control and Prevention has information on its web site at www.cdc.gov, as does WebMD, at www.webmd.com. Just type in the words *gallbladder disease* in the search box.

See Also: Medication, Diagnostic Testing, Inpatient Surgery, Pain Questions, and Pain After Surgery or a Procedure.

Getting Along in the Hospital: A Guide for Families

Ask, Ask, Ask

The hospital is a world unto itself, and unless you ask the right people the right questions, you are likely to feel lost, confused and frustrated.

Get to Know the Nurses

Nurses are licensed professionals who operate under standards and regulations; they are responsible for delivering quality care. Nurses play an important role in the healthcare environment. They are the front line of care, working with doctors and other healthcare professionals to coordinate quality patient care.

Nurses are responsible for the ongoing assessment and care of the patient. This makes them a good source of information about the patient's status.

The time when you are visiting your family member in the hospital may not coincide with the time your doctor makes rounds. Nurses working in the hospital do not always know when a doctor makes rounds, is in surgery, in the office, or in an emergency. If you do not see the doctor while you are visiting, remember that doctors usually work out of independent offices. Getting specific information and questions to a doctor may be done through the doctor's office. Leaving a cell phone number and work phone number is a good way to make it easier for the doctor to get back to you.

The following are tips for family survival during a hospital stay, which can be a stressful time.

Keep Visitors to a Minimum

In most ICU settings it is best to have no more than two visitors at a time. If there are more visitors they should wait in the waiting room, not in the hall outside the patient's room. It is important for all patients to have confidentiality; you can respect this by waiting in the waiting room.

Contact Person

Assign one family member as the contact person.

If a family has designated a spokesperson it will be easier to get information from and give information to the healthcare providers. That one person should be contacting family members to ensure that there are not extra phone calls to the hospital. Every time a nurse is called to the telephone, she is taken away from giving care to patients.

Questions

Keep a written list of questions that all family members have for the healthcare providers. It may be difficult to remember all the questions that you want to ask the doctors; having a written list of questions helps you to get the information that you need. The contact person should then pass on the information to other involved family members so all can be informed.

When a patient is hospitalized for a prolonged period and there are many specialists involved in his care, it may be difficult to get the whole picture. You may request a patient care conference where all the primary care givers can meet and agree on goals and plans. A patient care conference is a good time to discuss realistic outcomes for the patient. Advance Directives can be an important part of such discussions. Many people find that talking with the hospital chaplain, social worker or patient representative can provide instruction and support while making difficult decisions.

See also: Pain After Surgery or a Procedure, Who's Who in the Healthcare Setting, What's in the Chart, and Terminology.

Glaucoma Questions

What is glaucoma?

What causes glaucoma?

How is the diagnosis made?

What kind of glaucoma do I have?

What makes me vulnerable to glaucoma?

Are members of my family more likely to develop glaucoma?

How advanced is my glaucoma?

How quickly does the condition progress?

How can this be treated?

Can glaucoma be cured?

What are my treatment options?

Is laser surgery an option for me?

Is blindness always the end result of glaucoma?

How often should I have my eyes examined?

What can I do to protect my eyes?

Do you recommend that I take vitamin supplements such as antioxidants to protect my vision?

Where can I get more information about glaucoma?

TIP **The National Institutes of Health has a web site with information at www.nei.nih.gov, as does the Glaucoma Research Foundation, at www.glaucoma.org.**

See also: Medication.

Headache Questions

What type of headache am I having?

> **TIP** There are several categories of headache, including migraine, cluster and tension.

What causes this type of headache?

Should I have a CAT scan to rule out a more serious cause of my headaches?

Could a chronic sinus infection be causing these headaches?

> **TIP** Chronic sinus infections that do not have the typical symptoms can cause headaches and fatigue; this can best be diagnosed with a CAT scan.

Could my headaches be caused by unknown allergies?

> **TIP** Frequently, headaches are caused by allergies to food or environmental allergens. If you are having several headaches each week, you may benefit from thorough allergy testing.

Should I see an allergist to be tested?

Will I have blood tests to help rule out other health problems that may add to the headaches?

Should I become concerned if my headaches change (suddenly become accompanied by vomiting or difficulty seeing, for example)?

Can changes to my diet help ease my headaches?

Does exercise affect headaches?

Do you recommend that I try biofeedback to help control
my headaches?

What other methods do you recommend to relieve headache pain?

What medications do you recommend to control the pain
of headaches?

What should I be careful about when taking these medications?

> **TIP** Some over-the-counter pain relievers can cause liver damage when taken too
> frequently, and others may add to the problems of headaches when taken daily. Be
> sure to get specific instruction from your doctor about medications.

Do you have any helpful information that I can read
about headaches?

> **TIP** The American Council for Headache Education has information on its web site
> at www.achenet.org, as does WebMD, at www.webmd.com. Just type in the word
> *headache* in the search box.

See also: Medication, Emergency Room Article, and Emergency
Room Visit Questions.

Heart Attack (Myocardial Infarction) Questions

A heart attack (myocardial infarction) occurs when a part of the heart tissue (the myocardium) is deprived of oxygen for a period of time. This lack of oxygen causes the death of some cells and tissue in the heart muscle. The severity of the tissue loss depends on how much tissue was cut off from oxygen and for how long.

Is this heart attack severe?

How and when will you know how much damage is done to the heart?

What do the blood tests measure? How often will they be done?

> **TIP** Blood tests should be done immediately when a heart attack is suspected. These tests will measure damage done to the myocardium (heart muscle). The blood tests are usually done at 6- to 8-hour intervals. The first tests may be negative; damage may show in blood drawn 12 to 16 hours later.

What part of the heart is affected by this heart attack?

What is the treatment plan?

> **TIP** Frequently, an aspirin taken immediately after the signs of a heart attack begin can reduce the severity of the attack. Ask the emergency room staff if this is correct for you.

Will I need a cardiac catheterization?

> **TIP** In this procedure a catheter is inserted into an artery through a small incision in the groin. Intravenous dye is injected; the heart and surrounding blood vessels are viewed using an x-ray-like picture. This allows the cardiologist (medical doctor who is a heart specialist) to see your heart and the extent of the damage. The doctor may also be able to open closed arteries in your heart during this procedure.

What medication is being given to prevent more damage to the heart muscle?

Are anti-coagulants being given?

> **TIP** These are medications that are given to prevent abnormal clots from forming. They may be given to prevent a clot that can cause more damage to the heart.

How is my heart rate and blood pressure being controlled? How will these vital signs be monitored while I am in the hospital?

What is an acceptable heart rate and blood pressure in these circumstances?

Why is it important to keep the heart rate and blood pressure from being too high or too low?

How many days will I be in the hospital?

How long will it take me to recover from this?

Will I be in a cardiac rehabilitation program?

> **TIP** This is a program that you can attend on an outpatient basis. It may help you return to an active lifestyle and to understand heart disease.

What medications will I be taking (in the hospital and at home)?

Will I need to take medication for the rest of my life?

Is it necessary for me to stop smoking? Is secondhand smoke harmful to me?

Is alcohol harmful to me now?

Do I need to lose weight?

What is the best way for me to lose weight?

What exercise is safe for me to do?

When can I start to exercise/have sex/return to work?

Does this heart attack make it more likely that I will have another one?

Are there other health problems that I am likely to develop because of this heart attack?

> **TIP** People who have had significant damage to their heart are more vulnerable to congestive heart failure.

What can I do to avoid these health problems in the future?

Is there a web site or other resource that I can read to learn more about heart disease?

> **TIP** The American Heart Association has information on its web site at www.americanheart.org, as does WebMD, at www.webmd.com.

See also: Medication, Diagnostic Testing, Getting Along in the Hospital, Emergency Room Article, and Emergency Room Visit Questions.

Hiatal Hernia Questions

What is a hiatal hernia?

How did I develop this condition?

How is the diagnosis made?

What can I do to reduce the symptoms of this disease?

Do people with my condition usually require surgery?

What are the risks if my disease progresses?

Will antacids help or worsen my condition?

Are there any prescription medications that can help reduce
the symptoms?

Can I see a dietician to develop an eating plan that will help reduce
my symptoms?

Should I lose weight?

Will exercise help this condition?

Is there a web site where I can get more information?

> **TIP** The National Institutes for Health has information on its web site at
> www.niddk.nih.gov, as does WebMD, at www.webmd.com. Just type in *hiatal hernia*
> in the search box for information.

See also: Medication, and Outpatient Surgery.

High Blood Pressure/Hypertension

Blood Pressure is shown as two numbers, e.g., 110/62. The first or top number is the pressure that blood puts on the walls of your arteries when your heart pumps. The second or bottom number is the pressure on your arteries when your heart is in between beats.

It is important to keep your blood pressure in normal range. The American Heart Association guidelines say that if your blood pressure is higher than 140/90 it may be too high. It is a good idea to ask your doctor about what a good blood pressure is for you.

Many problems can be caused by high blood pressure. Remember that blood pressure measures the force on your arteries. If that force is even slightly higher than it should be for a long period of time, you may have a stroke (cerebral vascular accident). A stroke can be caused by a break in an artery that can cause bleeding in the brain.

Kidney damage can also be caused by high blood pressure. Over time, the small vessels that lead to your kidneys can be harmed if your blood pressure is high. This could mean that you will need to be on kidney dialysis.

Symptoms? There usually are not any symptoms—which is why high blood pressure has been called "the silent killer". Many people have stopped taking their prescribed blood pressure medication because they say they "feel great." This can be a tragic mistake and lead to death or disability. Patients should never stop taking blood pressure medication unless it is with the advice of their doctor.

Many doctors recommend that patients help to control their blood pressure by carefully changing their diet. Exercise can also help to lower blood pressure. Your doctor should be able to help advise you about what activities are safe for your situation.

Certain people are at a greater risk for high blood pressure. People with diabetes are at risk, as are overweight men and women. African-Americans have a greater risk of high blood pressure than other ethnic groups. People who smoke are at risk for blood pressure problems. Everyone should have his blood pressure checked and consult a doctor about this important health issue.

More information about high blood pressure can be found on the American Heart Association's web site at www.americanheart.org.

See also: High Blood Pressure Questions, and Medication.

High Blood Pressure Questions

What should my blood pressure be?

Does my blood pressure indicate that I have a serious health problem?

What are the best ways to control my blood pressure?

Does the food that I eat affect my blood pressure?

Does my weight or level of activity affect my blood pressure?

Will smoking cigarettes or cigars affect my blood pressure?

What problems can my blood pressure cause for me? Why is it important to control my blood pressure?

If taking medication:

How does this medication lower/control my blood pressure?

Is this the usual dose for this medication?

Are there side effects to this medication?

Can I stop taking this medication if I cannot tolerate the side effects?

Can I stop taking this medication if I feel well?

TIP Blood pressure medication usually needs to be taken every day—it can be very dangerous to stop taking it without the advice of your doctor.

If I cannot afford all of my medication, are there ones that are most important to take?

How will this medication work with my other medications?

Can I take vitamins or other supplements with this medication?

Where can I get more information about this condition?

TIP The American Heart Association has information on its web site at www.americanheart.org, as does WebMD, at www.webmd.com.

See also: Medication, and High Blood Pressure/Hypertension.

Hip Fracture Questions

What part of the hip is fractured?

Can you show me a picture of the bones involved?

Can you show me on the x-ray?

What caused my hip to break?

> **TIP** Frequently people fall and break a hip, yet the fall may not have caused the fracture. The actual fracture may have happened first, and then the fall. If you did fall, it is important to know WHY you fell.

Do I have osteoporosis?

> **TIP** See Osteoporosis.

Will I need surgery?

Will I be in traction?

While I wait for surgery, and after surgery, will I have physical therapy?

> **TIP** It is important to properly exercise the unaffected leg and your arms to prevent loss of muscle tone and to help with your recovery.

What measures will be taken to ensure that I do not get bedsores while I am less able to move in bed?

What is my risk for getting a blood clot?

Do I have health problems that may complicate surgery and recovery?

What can I do to avoid another hip fracture?

Does my nutritional status make me vulnerable to having a fracture?

Who will help me with plans for discharge from the hospital?

> **TIP** It is very important to plan for your discharge immediately. You may need equipment and other help when you are discharged; the hospital may have a discharge planner to assist you.

Do you have any information that I can read about hip fractures?

> **TIP** The American Academy of Orthopaedic Surgeons has a web site with information at www.aaos.org, as does WebMD, at www.webmd.com. Just type in *hip fracture* in the search box.

See also: Orthopedic Surgery, Pain After Surgery or a Procedure, Pain Questions, Getting Along in the Hospital, and Anesthesia.

Hospice Care Questions

Hospice care is designed to care for patients who are at the end of their lives. Its purpose is to treat pain and to alleviate symptoms, rather than curing the disease. While hospice care is not directed toward curing the disease, it also does not cause death to happen sooner. Healthcare professionals who specialize in hospice care seek to help patients and their families experience the patient's death with a sense of dignity and peace.

Who determines that the patient is appropriate for hospice?

Where is hospice care given?

> **TIP** Hospice care is usually designed to help the patient stay at home. But hospice care can be given in certain hospitals, nursing homes, and other settings.

What is the difference in the care that the patient receives in hospice care and that received in a traditional medical approach?

Does being a hospice patient mean that nothing is being done to help the patient?

What are the specific services that the hospice patient and family receive?

Who are the members of the hospice team that will work with the patient and family?

How often will the patient receive home visits from the doctor and nurses?

> **TIP** Because hospice patients are quite ill, home visits are an important part of hospice care.

While receiving hospice care, can the patient continue with his regular physician?

> **TIP** Generally the hospice physician directs the care for hospice patients. Some programs may accommodate the request to work together with your doctor.

Can hospice patients be treated by a physical therapist?

> **TIP** Some hospice patients benefit from physical therapy because it can help them remain more physically capable. Physical therapy can also help some types of pain problems, improve mobility and prevent bedsores.

If the patient changes his mind about hospice care or his condition greatly improves, can he decide to discontinue hospice care?

Is it necessary to have Advance Directives or a medical power of attorney to be a hospice patient?

Can hospice patients still receive IV fluids, tube feedings, antibiotics, and pain medication?

> **TIP** Each hospice may have slightly different philosophies of care regarding these options. Most respect the preferences of the patient and family regarding these specifics of treatment, as long as it is understood that the goal of treatment is not to cure the underlying disease. The goal of hospice care is to treat the patient's symptoms and to maximize the comfort for the patient's remaining days.

If a hospice patient is at home and suddenly becomes much more ill or experiences sudden severe symptoms, such as difficulty breathing, should the family call 911 or other emergency medical help?

Where can I learn more about hospice care?

> **TIP** The Hospice Foundation has a web site with information at www.hospicefoundation.org, as does the National Hospice and Palliative Care Organization, at www.nhpco.org.

See also: Advance Directives/End of Life Decisions, Pain Questions, and Pain After Surgery or a Procedure.

Hypothyroid
(Low Levels of Thyroid Hormone)
Questions

What is the function of thyroid hormone?

What tests are done to confirm the diagnosis of hypothyroidism?

Is the diagnosis made based on blood tests and on the symptoms that I report?

Does my physical exam show signs of hypothyroidism?

> **TIP** This condition is usually accompanied by specific symptoms and can also cause enlarging of the heart, gastrointestinal problems and reproductive problems.

Will I need to take medication to correct this imbalance in thyroid hormone?

Will I need to take this medication for the rest of my life?

How do you know the dose of medication is right for me?

Will I need to come back to have my thyroid hormone levels checked after I start to take the medication?

Are my other hormone levels normal?

> **TIP** If you have inadequate levels of estrogen or testosterone, or are insulin resistant, you may have symptoms of hypothyroidism. Your symptoms may not improve if your other hormone levels are not in balance; it is reasonable to ask to have them checked, because they all work as a team.

Are there other health problems that can be mistaken for hypothyroidism?

Should I see an endocrinologist?

> **TIP** This is a medical doctor who specializes in the diagnosis and treatment of hormone-related problems, such as hypothyroidism.

What changes/improvement in my condition will the medication provide?

How soon should I notice the improvement?

If there are no improvements, why should I continue to take the medication?

Are there changes that I can make in my lifestyle instead of taking medication?

What changes should I make in my diet?

> **TIP** Be cautious about very low-calorie diets—they can increase your symptoms of fatigue. Diets that severely restrict fat and protein may also increase your symptoms of dry skin, brittle hair and nails. There are many books about nutrition that you can access at the library or bookstore. Your doctor may be able to recommend a resource for good, balanced nutrition.

How can exercise help this condition?

Is there a web site where I can read more about hypothyroidism?

> **TIP** WebMD has information on its web site at www.webmd.com. Type in *thyroid problems* in the search box.

See also: Medication, Depression, and Diagnostic Testing.

Hysterectomy Questions

Why do I need this procedure?

Is this a common reason to need a hysterectomy?

> **TIP** According to the Centers for Disease Control, the three conditions most frequently associated with hysterectomy are: fibroid tumors, endometriosis, and uterine prolapse.

Whom do you recommend that I see for a second opinion?

> **TIP** It is very reasonable for you to seek a second opinion about such an important issue—you do not need to feel that you are being disloyal to your doctor to ask for a second opinion.

Is there a nonsurgical treatment that I could try?

What would happen if I delay having surgery?

What method would you use for surgery?

> **TIP** Hysterectomies can be performed either vaginally or abdominally. Usually the vaginal approach requires less healing time after surgery.

Will my ovaries be removed?

What are the advantages/disadvantages to having my ovaries removed?

What hormones will I need to have replaced after surgery?

> **TIP** Both the uterus and the ovaries play a role in hormone function in your body. You may want to consider hormone replacement therapy after surgery.

What changes will my body go through after this surgery?

Can you recommend reading that I should do to educate myself on this procedure and its consequences/side effects?

How will my pain be controlled in the hospital?

TIP See Pain Questions, and Inpatient Surgery.

How long will I be in the hospital?

How long will I need to be off of work?

Will I have a higher risk of heart disease and osteoporosis after surgery?

Am I likely to experience depression as a result of the hormonal changes in my body after surgery?

Is this the course of treatment you would recommend for a member of your family?

Where can I get more information about hysterectomy surgery?

TIP The Centers for Disease Control and Prevention has information on its web site at www.cdc.gov, as does WebMD, at www.webmd.com. Just type in *hysterectomy* in the search box.

See also: Inpatient Surgery, Pain Questions, Menopause, and Medication.

Immunizations Questions

What is the immunization schedule for my child?

How do immunizations affect my child's immune system?

What are the risks if I choose not to follow the immunization schedule?

> **TIP** Some immunizations that are usually combined (e.g., the MMR) can be given at separate times if you request it.

Are there additional immunizations that I should consider that are not required?

> **TIP** Currently, the chicken pox (varicella) vaccine is not universally required, although the American Academy of Pediatrics recommends it.

Should I pre-medicate my child with acetaminophen or ibuprofen before getting immunizations?

What reactions should I watch for after having immunizations?

How significant is the risk of seizure after having immunizations?

Will giving acetaminophen or ibuprofen before my child develops a fever help reduce the risk of seizure?

What comfort measures do you recommend to help make this a less stressful event for my child and me?

Do you recommend that my child and/or I have the flu vaccine every year in the fall?

If I have not had the hepatitis B vaccine series, should I get it now?

Are there other vaccinations that you recommend for adults or older children?

> **TIP** If you or your older child have not had chicken pox, you may want to ask your doctor if she recommends the varicella vaccine.

What is the evidence about autism and immunizations?

Do you have any reading material about immunizations, or can you recommend a web site where I can learn more about this subject?

> **TIP** The Centers for Disease Control and Prevention has information on its web site at www.cdc.gov/nip. The American Academy of Pediatrics also has information on its web site at www.aap.org.

Influenza (Flu) Questions

What causes the flu?

How can I tell if I have the flu instead of a cold?

Why is the flu dangerous?

> **TIP** According to the Centers for Disease Control, influenza is a leading cause of death among older Americans.

How can I avoid getting the flu?

> **TIP** The most effective way to avoid getting sick is to practice good hand washing. Wash your hands for 15 seconds using soap and running water before you eat, after using the washroom, and when around people who have colds or flu symptoms.

Should I get a flu vaccination every year?

> **TIP** The Centers for Disease Control recommends that certain people at risk for the complications from flu get vaccinated, usually in the fall months. People at risk include those with compromised immune symptoms and older people.

What are the risks to getting vaccinated?

Will getting vaccinated give me flu symptoms for the next few days?

If I get the flu, should I take antibiotics?

> **TIP** Viruses cause the flu; they are not effectively treated with antibiotics. Taking antibiotics when they are not effective can make you susceptible to other health problems that your doctor can explain.

What can I do to make myself feel better if I get the flu?

What are the signs that I need to see the doctor if I get the flu?

What are the signs that I should go to the emergency room
for treatment?

Are there changes to my diet that I should make to avoid getting the flu
or to strengthen my immune system?

Where can I learn more about the flu?

> **TIP** The Centers for Disease Control and Prevention has information on its web site
> at www.cdc.gov. Just go to Health Topics under the letter *F* for flu. WebMD also
> has information on its web site at www.webmd.com. Just type in the word *flu* in the
> search box.

See also: Immunization, Emergency Room Article, Emergency Room
Visit Questions, and Medication.

Inpatient Surgery Questions

Inpatient surgery is surgery requiring admission to the hospital for 24 hours or more.

Who will be performing the surgery?

> **TIP** As the patient, it is reasonable for you to ask who specifically will be involved in your case. In some hospitals resident doctors may be involved in surgical procedures.

Do I need preoperative blood tests? Where can this be done?

What should I do the day and evening before the surgery?

Should I take my regular medications, including aspirin or vitamins, the day of surgery?

Do I need to be NPO (nothing by mouth: nothing to eat or drink for a certain period of time) the evening before the surgery?

What time should I arrive for the surgery?

How long will I be in the holding room before surgery?

What time will the surgery actually begin?

What are the most common complications related to this surgery?

What has been this surgeon's experience with complications?

Does my past medical history create risk for complications?

What specific measures are taken to avoid complications?

Will I need to receive a blood transfusion?
Can my family members or I donate blood for my surgery?

TIP This must be done in advance and requires a doctor's order.

What type of anesthesia will be used? Do I have options for different types of anesthesia?

Who will be giving me the anesthesia?

What types of monitoring devices will be used during the surgery?

How long will I be in surgery?

What will happen immediately after the surgery?

Will I go to the recovery room? How long should I expect to be in the recovery room?

Will the doctor see me in the recovery room to be sure that my pain is controlled?

Will my family members be informed if there is a delay in the process?

How soon after the surgery will my family members be able to see me?

Who will keep my family informed during the procedure?

TIP Many hospitals have a nurse liaison to keep family members informed during surgery.

What will I be given to relieve pain after surgery?

What level of pain do patients generally experience immediately after surgery? The next day? One week later?

Will a pain specialist see me?

After the recovery room, will I be taken to a regular hospital room or the intensive care unit?

Will I need oxygen or a ventilator after surgery?

Will I need a laxative or other bowel program (promotes regularity to avoid the complication of constipation) after surgery?

What will I have in or on my body when I wake up after surgery?

> **TIP** You may have: **breathing tube, IV catheter, urine catheter, chest tube, staples or stitches, heart monitor, oxygen, nasogastric tube, pulse oximeter, surgical stockings.**

Will I need blood tests or x-rays after surgery?

Should I expect swelling after surgery?

What activities are expected of me after surgery?

When will I start getting out of the bed to a chair?

Why is coughing, deep breathing and repositioning so important to my recovery process?

Will a dietician be involved in my care?

How long will I be in the hospital?

Does the hospital have recommendations for overnight accommodations for my family?

Do you allow family members to stay overnight with the patient?

> **TIP** It may be appropriate for you to have someone at the bedside while you are in the hospital. This is individual for each case. Family members should be careful to take care of themselves as well as be concerned for the patient during this stressful time. It may be necessary to ask to speak with the nurse manager or patient representative to make arrangements to have a family member at the bedside overnight.

Will I need someone to stay with me at home?

Will I need to make special arrangements for home prior to discharge?

Will a social worker or discharge planner be involved in my care?

When can I start my normal activities (exercising, driving, sexual activity, etc.)?

When can I go back to work?

What can I do to improve my recovery process (diet, exercise, stop smoking, or vitamins)?

Where can I get more information about this surgery?

> **TIP** The Surgery Channel web site has information at www.surgerychannel.com, as does WebMD, at www.webmd.com. Just type in the name of the surgery in the search box.

See also: Pain Questions, Advance Directives/End-of-Life Decisions, Who's Who in the Healthcare Setting, and Getting Along in the Hospital.

Kidney Disease (Renal Disease) Questions

How did I develop this condition?

What functions did my kidneys perform that they are unable to perform now?

Is this condition reversible?

What other problems might I experience as a result of my kidney disease? (Examples are skin discoloration, itching and dryness, congestive heart failure, anemia and high blood pressure)

Will I need to restrict the amount and type of fluid I drink every day?

Can I see a dietician to help me with my new diet?

Why is it important to follow a new diet?

What role do dietary electrolytes have in kidney disease?

Is there anything I can do now to stop this from getting worse?

What new medications will I be taking?

How will these work with my other medications?

What medications or dietary supplements should I avoid taking?

What changes to my body are important to notify you about
(such as sudden weight gain, unusual fatigue, swollen legs or difficulty
breathing)?

When should I go to the emergency room?

What are the most important things my family and friends need to
know about my disease to help me stay healthy?

Will I need peritoneal dialysis or hemodialysis?

Is it possible I will need a kidney transplant?

Is there a web site or book I can read to get more information about
kidney disease?

> **TIP** WebMD has a web site with information at www.webmd.com, or the National
> Kidney Foundation, at www.kidney.org

See also: Medication, Transplant Surgery, and High
Blood Pressure.

Kidney Stone Questions

A common symptom is pain in the flank region (lower back and side of abdomen). The pain may be constant or come and go in a cramping manner. The pain may be very severe. Urinary frequency, nausea and vomiting may also occur.

What are kidney stones?

What causes this condition?

What tests are done to diagnose kidney stones?

> **TIP** Frequently an analysis of your urine is required; the doctor may also order an x-ray or CAT scan. A blood test may be done.

Can anything be done to remove the stone?

How long will it take for the stone to pass out through my urine?

Is it painful when the stone passes?

Will I need to be in the hospital to get adequate pain control?

> **TIP** Frequently, kidney stones are diagnosed in the emergency room. Typically, patients are given IV fluids and sent home with pain medication and a strainer to strain their urine until the stone passes. There are patients who need to be admitted to the hospital to obtain adequate pain control. You may discuss the options with your doctor.

Am I more likely to get kidney stones in the future?

What can I do to prevent kidney stones?

Are there changes in my eating habits that I should make to help my overall health and to prevent kidney stones?

What medications will I be prescribed to alleviate the pain?

Do I need an antibiotic medication?

What symptoms would indicate that this is becoming a more serious condition?

Do you have information that I can read about kidney stones?

> **TIP** The National Institutes for Health has information on its web site at www.niddk.nih.gov, as does WebMD, at: www.webmd.com. Just type in *kidney stone* in the search boxes.

See also: Medication, Emergency Room Article, Emergency Room Visit Questions, Diagnostic Testing, Pain Questions, and Pain After Surgery or Procedure.

Lupus
(Systemic Erythematosus Lupus)
Questions

What tests are done to diagnose lupus?

May I have a copy of my blood tests?

TIP It is a good idea to keep your own file of your medical records and test results.

What causes this condition?

Does this always get worse over time?

What is specifically happening in my body as a result of lupus?

TIP Lupus affects many body systems. It will be helpful to have an understanding of how this complex disease works.

What is remission and how does it affect lupus patients?

Am I likely to develop arthritis?

How does lupus affect my heart?

Am I more likely to develop heart disease?

TIP Many people with lupus develop heart problems.

What problems can lupus cause for my kidneys?

How will I be tested for heart and kidney problems? How often?

What specifically can I do to avoid problems with my heart
and kidneys?

Should I see a specialist to manage the lupus before it
becomes severe?

> **TIP** Rhuematologists are medical doctors who specialize in the treatment of
> patients with this type of disease.

Should I change my diet?

> **TIP** Good nutrition may not be a cure for lupus, but having a balanced, healthy diet
> will help your overall health and may help you to avoid further problems.

Should I lose weight?

> **TIP** Excess weight will put additional strain on your joints, heart and other body
> systems that are already stressed by lupus.

What sort of activity/exercise should I be doing to help make
myself stronger?

Are there activities that I should avoid?

> **TIP** Some people with lupus are very sensitive to sunlight; this is not true for all
> people with lupus—ask your doctor if you should avoid being in the sun.

Is my lupus likely to get worse if I become pregnant?

What medications will I take to help with the symptoms of lupus?

> **TIP** The medications given for lupus are to manage symptoms rather than to cure
> the disease.

What are the advantages/disadvantages to these medications?

If I take steroids to help with the symptoms of lupus, am I more
vulnerable to heart and bone problems later?

Are there medications that I should NOT take?

> **TIP** There are some antibiotics, and other medications that may exacerbate lupus symptoms—ask your doctor for a list of these medications.

Am I at risk for abnormal bleeding and infections?

How will I be monitored for these problems?

Is there a support group I can attend, or reading that I can do, to get more information about lupus?

> **TIP** The Lupus Foundation of America has information on its web site at www.lupus.org, as does the Arthritis Foundation, at www.arthritis.org. Just type in *lupus* in the search box.

See also: Medication, and Diagnostic Testing.

Medication Questions

When a doctor prescribes a medication for you, it is usually after careful consideration of what you need for your condition. However, even with the most trusted doctor, you should have your questions answered before you begin to take a new medication. The following is a list of suggested questions that are appropriate for many situations, whether the medication is an antibiotic or a complicated heart medication. Remember that your pharmacist may also be able to give you important information regarding your medication and should be regarded as an important part of your healthcare team.

How does this medication help me?

Is this the usual dose for someone in my situation?

Do you usually prescribe this medicine for patients with my health situation?

How long will I need to take this medicine?

Is this an expensive medication?

Is there an alternative that may be less expensive?

How long has this medication been on the market?

What will happen if I miss a dose or an entire day of the medication?

> **TIP** Some medications such as antibiotics may lose their effectiveness if you miss a day. Other medications are so important that your health may be in danger if you even miss one dose.

How will this medicine interact with other medicines that I am taking?

> **TIP** Keep a written list of your current medications with you at all times in your purse or wallet.

Can I drink alcohol while taking this medicine?

> **TIP** Some medicines can have a dangerous interaction with alcohol, even with beer and wine. Some medications may not be effective if you drink alcohol while taking them.

Will this medicine have undesirable side effects? Will it affect my sleeping? Appetite? Sex drive?

What can I do if I have bad side effects?

Will the medicine make me urinate often?

Will it make me constipated or have diarrhea?

Will my vitamins or herbs interact with this medication?

Do you have additional information that I can read about this medication?

> **TIP** You may be able to obtain more information on the Internet about specific medications. The WebMD web site has information on various medications at www.webmd.com.

See also: What to Ask at Your Next Doctor's Appointment, Emergency Room Article, and Emergency Room Visit Questions.

Menopause Questions

How will I know that I am entering menopause?

Can you take a blood test to measure the hormone levels that I have at this time?

> **TIP** Knowing what your hormone levels are will allow you to keep track over time. It will also help your doctor know whether you truly are in menopause or if there is another problem causing your symptoms. It will also help in the process of discovering what levels you need if you choose hormone replacement therapy.

What changes in my body will I notice over the next few months?
Can I get pregnant during menopause?

Does the fact that my hormone levels are falling mean that I am susceptible to some diseases?

> **TIP** There is evidence that estrogen protects women from heart disease as well as osteoporosis (thinning of the bones).

What can I do to help prevent these health problems after menopause?

What should I do if I feel heart palpitations or chest pain?

Can increasing my exercise help to prevent some of the problems of menopause?

Are there changes in my diet that I should make now?

How important is it that I stop smoking during menopause?

Will you recommend that I have my bone density tested?

> **TIP** Many women have early stages of osteoporosis without knowing it.

How frequently should I have a mammogram?

Do you recommend hormone replacement therapy (HRT), for me?

If you do recommend HRT, are you going to prescribe real hormones to replace what I have lost?

> **TIP** There are many different forms of hormone replacement therapy; some are synthetic hormones, and some are real hormones. Ask your doctor to explain the benefits of the specific type of hormone that is prescribed.

Are there non-prescription medications that I can take to help relieve the effects of menopause?

Should I see an endocrinologist (a medical doctor whose specialty is how hormones affect the body)?

Is there a book or web site that you can recommend so that I can get more informed about this important stage of my life?

> **TIP** The Federal Consumer Information Center (1-888-878-3256) offers a booklet about hormone replacement therapy, and author Christiane Northrup, MD, has several books on the market about menopause and women's health issues. The WebMD web site has information about menopause at www.webmd.com. Just type in the word *menopause* in the search box.

See also: Hypothyroid, Osteoporosis, and Medication.

Mitral Valve Prolapse (MVP or Heart Murmur) Questions

What is Mitral Valve Prolapse?

How is the diagnosis made?

Should I have an echocardiogram?

Should I have an EKG?

Is this a dangerous condition?

How do you determine whether mine is a serious problem or not?

Should I be referred to a cardiologist (heart specialist)?

What are the symptoms of a heart murmur?

Will I experience chest pain as a result of having MVP?

If I have chest pain should I go to the emergency room or call my doctor's office?

Does having MVP mean that I have an irregular heartbeat?

Does MVP make me more vulnerable to having a heart attack?

Can drinking more water decrease the symptoms of MVP?

Should I lose weight or make other nutritional changes to improve my overall health?

Will exercise improve my MVP?

Do I need to take any new medications to help my MVP?

Should I take any vitamins or nutritional supplements?

Am I allowed to be a blood donor?

Should I take antibiotics prior to having dental work done?

> **TIP** With certain kinds of heart murmurs, there is an increased risk of developing a serious heart infection after dental work or surgery. Be sure to clarify this with your doctor.

Can you give me further information about MVP or refer me to a web site where I can learn more about this condition?

> **TIP** The American Heart Association has more information on their web site at www.americanheart.org, as does WebMD, at www.Webmd.com. Just type in the letters *MVP* in the search boxes.

See also: Medication, Emergency Room Article, and Emergency Room Visit Questions.

Mononucleosis (Mono) Questions

What causes mono?

How is it spread?

Should I avoid being around other people to avoid spreading this infection?

How is the diagnosis made?

> **TIP** The diagnosis is usually made after a physical exam and a blood test.

Do you recommend that the people with whom I have been in close contact to get tested for mono?

What can I do to prevent this from spreading to the people with whom I live?

> **TIP** You may want to use the sterilizing option on your dishwasher, if you have one.

What symptoms of mono do I have?

Will I need a blood test?

When will I get the results of the test?

What should I do until the test results are known?

How is mono treated?

Will I need an antibiotic?

TIP Mononucleosis is a viral infection and therefore is not treated with antibiotics.

Can mono be dangerous?

What can I do to avoid complications from mono?

What can I do to help myself feel better?

Should I make specific changes in my diet?

Do you recommend that I take vitamins or other nutritional supplements?

Are there activities that I should avoid while I have mono?

How long does mono last?

Can I get mono more than once?

Do you have more information that I can read about mononucleosis?

TIP The Centers for Disease Control and Prevention has a web site with information at www.cdc.gov; look under *Health Topics A-Z.* And WebMD has information on its web site at www.webmd.com. Just type in *mono* in the search box.

See also: Medication, and Diagnostic Testing.

Multiple Sclerosis (MS) Questions

How is this diagnosis made?

> **TIP** There is not one definitive test for MS; there are usually several symptoms that lead to the diagnosis. Many doctors recommend an MRI. This allows the doctor to see if there is damage to the myelin sheath surrounding certain nerve fibers.

Which of my symptoms lead to the diagnosis of MS?

Could these symptoms be from another cause other than MS?

> **TIP** There are other conditions that may present with symptoms similar to MS, such as Lyme disease.

Will I need a lumbar puncture (spinal tap)?

How does examining cerebral spinal fluid aid in the diagnosis of MS?

Is this a fatal disease?

Does MS always get worse over time?

Will I have periods of remission (times when the MS symptoms are not as noticeable)?

What treatments are effective to control MS?

Is there a cure?

Will steroids be part of my treatment?

Would I benefit from making changes to my diet?

Do you recommend that I take vitamins or other supplements to help my overall health?

Should I lose weight?

> **TIP** If you are carrying excess weight, the symptoms of fatigue may be worse for you.

Is it important for me to exercise regularly? What is the best type of exercise for me?

What is the likely progression of this disease over the next few months and years?

Am I going to have cognitive problems (difficulty thinking, memory problems)?

Am I likely to develop depression?

Am I vulnerable to other health problems as a result of MS?

Can I become pregnant?

Will pregnancy worsen the condition?

Will I experience problems with bladder control?

Will I experience sexual dysfunction?

Are there support groups, books or web sites that I can consult to learn more about MS?

> **TIP** There are several organizations that provide information about MS. WebMD has information on its web site at www.webmd.com. Just type in *MS* in the search box.

See also: Medication, Depression, and Diagnostic Testing.

Nutritional Support

When you are sick, and especially after surgery, nutrition is an important part of the healing process. A dietician may be involved in many aspects of the healthcare process. A dietician may be consulted to speak with you about your present diet and make suggestions for changes, offer meal plans, and help you to make the best food choices for your condition. Dieticians also work closely with physicians to choose the appropriate type of tube feeding as well as IV nutrition (called total parentaral nutrition).

Special Diets
A physician must order any food provided to a patient in the hospital. There are many types of diets that can help to balance the body for a variety of conditions and circumstances.

Enteral Feeding or Tube Feeding
This is liquid nutrition fed via a tube in the patient's stomach or intestine. The feeding tube may be inserted down a patient's nose and into the stomach or, for long-term feeding, a tube will be surgically inserted through the skin into the stomach. Patients who are unable to eat due to a ventilator, extensive surgery or trauma may be fed this way.

Intravenous Feeding or Total Parentaral Nutrition (TPN)
This is specially formulated solution given to patients via an IV catheter. TPN is dramatically different from regular IV fluid because it provides complex nutritional support.

Cardiac Diet
Restricted in fat and sodium.

Clear Liquid
Gelatins, broth, coffee, tea, and some juices.

Diabetic Diet
Calorie-controlled for the special needs of the diabetic patient, often following the guidelines of the American Diabetic Association. This diet balances the intake of carbohydrates, fats and proteins in specific proportions.

Renal Diet
Restricted in protein, potassium and sodium content.

Soft Diet
Foods that require a small amount of chewing, such as soups, mashed potatoes, pureed foods or ground meats.

General Diet
An unrestricted diet; patients can choose from a variety of foods and calorie levels.

After Surgery
When a person undergoes anesthesia, an effect of the anesthetic agents results in a temporary slowing of normal bowel function. This means that the bowels stop contracting as normal. If you eat regular food soon after general anesthesia it may not be able to pass from the stomach into the intestine. This can cause you to vomit. After most surgeries you are given broth and other liquids. The doctors and nurses will listen to your abdomen to hear bowel sounds. If your bowel is "awake" there will be bowel sounds, and you may be allowed to eat.

General anesthesia may cause nausea even if you do not eat or drink. See Anesthesia for more information.

More information about nutrition and health can be found on the WebMD web site at www.webmd.com. The Food and Nutrition Information Center, in cooperation with the United States Department of Agriculture, has information at www.nal.usda.gov/fnic.

Organ and Tissue Donation Questions

This can be a sensitive subject for a lot of people. Talk with your doctor about donation to learn more. There are over 79,000 people waiting for organ and tissue transplants. Each day 15 people die while waiting for a transplant. It is important to let your family members know what your wishes are regarding organ donation.

What types of organs and tissues can be donated?

Are there conditions that would exclude me from being able to donate?

How do I let people know that I want to be an organ donor?

Can my family prevent me from being an organ donor after I die?

Will it affect the quality or type of care that I receive in the hospital if I am a declared organ donor?

Can I choose what organs to donate?

Will organ donation mutilate my body?

Will I be able to have an open casket at my funeral?

Is there a web site or other information that I can read about organ donation?

> **TIP** The United States Department of Health and Human Services has a web site with information at www.organdonor.gov, as does WebMD, at www.webmd.com. Just type in *organ donation* in the search box.

See also: Advance Directives/End-of-Life Decisions.

Orthopedic Surgery Questions

Who will be performing the surgery?

> **TIP** As the patient, it is reasonable for you to ask who specifically will be involved in your case.

Do I need preoperative blood tests? Where can this be done?

What should I do the day before the surgery?

Should I take my regular medications, including aspirin or vitamins, the day of surgery?

Do I need to be NPO (nothing by mouth: nothing to eat or drink for a certain period of time) the evening before the surgery?

What time should I arrive for the surgery?

How long will I be in the holding room before surgery?

What time will the surgery actually begin?

Will I need to receive a blood transfusion?

Can my family members or I donate blood for my surgery?

> **TIP** This must be done in advance and requires a doctor's order.

What are the most common complications related to this procedure?

Are air and fat emboli a concern for this surgery?

> **TIP** Ask your doctor to explain this complication.

What has been this surgeon's experience with complications?

Does my past medical history create risk for complications?

What specific measures are taken to avoid complications?

What type of anesthesia will be used? Do I have options for different types of anesthesia?

Who will be giving me the anesthesia?

> **TIP** You may ask to speak with the anesthesiologist or nurse anesthetist before the day of surgery.

What types of monitoring devices will be used during the surgery?

How long will the surgery take?

What will happen immediately after the surgery?

Will I go to the recovery room? How long should I expect to be in the recovery room?

Will the surgeon see me in the recovery room to be sure that my pain is controlled?

How soon after surgery will my family member be able to see me?

Who will keep my family informed during the surgery?

> **TIP** Many hospitals have a nurse liaison to keep family members informed during surgery.

What will I be given to relieve pain after surgery?

What level of pain do patients generally experience immediately after surgery? The next day? One week later?

Will a pain specialist see me?

After the Recovery Room will I be taken to a regular hospital room or the intensive care unit?

Will I need a laxative or other bowel program (promotes regularity to avoid the complication of constipation) after surgery?

How will I go to the washroom?

Will I be given medication to prevent blood clots?

What are the precautions that I need to take while taking this medication?

What will I have in or on my body when I wake up (such as IVs, urine catheter, staples or stitches, heart monitor, oxygen, nasogastric tube, pulse oximetry or surgical stockings)?

Should I expect swelling after surgery?

> **TIP** Ice therapy may help relieve pain and swelling. Ask you doctor about this.

How will my circulation and nerve function be monitored after surgery?

> **TIP** Numbness and tingling of the affected body part could be important symptoms to report to your doctor or nurse.

What activities are expected of me after surgery?

Will I need physical therapy after surgery?

Will I need any orthopedic equipment (such as a walker) or a special hospital bed?

When will I need to start getting out of the bed to a chair?

Why is coughing, deep breathing and repositioning so important to my recovery process?

How long will I be in the hospital?

Will I require a special diet?

Will I speak with a dietician?

Does the hospital have recommendations for overnight accommodations for my family?

Do you allow family members to stay overnight with the patient?

> **TIP** It may be appropriate for you to have someone at the bedside while you are in the hospital. This is individual for each case. Family members should be careful to take care of themselves as well as be concerned for the patient during this stressful time. It may be necessary to ask to speak with the nurse manager or patient representative to make arrangements to have a family member at the bedside overnight.

Will I need someone to stay with me at home?

Will I need to make special arrangements for home prior to discharge?

Will a social worker or discharge planner be involved in my care?

When can I start my normal activities such as exercising, driving and sexual activity?

When can I go back to work?

What can I do to improve my recovery process (such as changes in my diet, exercising or stopping smoking)?

Where can I get more information about this type of surgery?

TIP **The American Academy of Orthopedic Surgeons has information on its web site at www.aaos.org, as does WebMD, at www.webmd.com. Just type in the name of the surgery in the search box.**

See also: Pain Questions, Advance Directives/End-of-Life Decisions, Who's Who in the Healthcare Setting, and Getting Along in the Hospital.

Osteoporosis Questions

What causes osteoporosis?

Should I have a bone density scan?

What factors make me vulnerable to osteoporosis?

Why is this a possibly dangerous condition?

Can osteoporosis cause neck and head pain?

> **TIP** This condition can affect the bones in your neck.

What can I do to help increase the strength of my bones?

Are weight bearing exercises or aerobic exercises better for my bone strength?

Should I work with a physical therapist?

What changes in my nutrition should I make?

What supplements should I be taking?

Would hormone replacement therapy help improve this condition?

Can you recommend a book or web site where I can learn more about osteoporosis?

> **TIP** The Centers for Disease Control and Prevention has a web site with information at www.cdc.gov. WebMD has information on its web site at www.webmd.com. Just type in *osteoporosis* in the search box.

See also: Medication, and Diagnostic Testing.

Outpatient Surgery Questions

Many hospitals refer to this as ambulatory or same-day surgery. This includes procedures that allow the patient to go home within 23 hours of admission.

Who will be performing the surgery?

> **TIP** As the patient, it is reasonable for you to ask who specifically will be involved in your case.

How many of these surgeries do you perform each year?

Do I need preoperative blood tests? Where can this be done?

What should I do the day before the surgery?

Do I need to be NPO (nothing by mouth: nothing to eat or drink for a certain period of time) the evening before the procedure?

Should I take my regular medications, including aspirin or vitamins, the day of surgery?

What time should I arrive for the surgery?

Is there a specific place where I should park?

How long will I be in the holding room before surgery?

What time will the surgery actually begin?

What are the most common complications related to this procedure?

What has been this surgeon's experience with complications?

Does my past medical history create risk for complications?

What specific measures are taken to avoid complications?

What circumstances would make overnight admission to the hospital necessary?

What type of anesthesia will be used? Do I have options for different types of anesthesia?

Who will be giving me the anesthesia?

> **TIP** You may ask to speak to the anesthesiologist or nurse anesthetist before the day of the surgery.

What types of monitoring devices will be used during the surgery?

How long will the surgery take?

What will happen immediately after the surgery?

Will the doctor check on me in the recovery room to be sure that my pain is controlled?

How soon after surgery will my family member be able to see me?

Who will keep my family informed during the procedure?

> **TIP** Many hospitals have a nurse liaison to keep family members informed during surgery.

When can I go home after the surgery?

What will I be given to relieve pain after surgery?

What level of pain do patients generally experience immediately after surgery? The next day? One week later?
Is it possible to have my postoperative prescriptions filled before

the procedure?

> **TIP** Be sure you have your pharmacy's phone number with you.

Will I need to arrange transportation home?

Will I need a family member or a friend with me when I return home?

What do I need to know about the recovery process at home?

If I experience problems after I return home, what number should I call?

> **TIP** Problems may include unexpected bleeding or pain not relieved with the pain medication.

When can I start my normal activities, such as exercising, driving and sexual activity?

When can I go back to work?

How many follow-up visits do I need? Will I be seeing the doctor or someone else?

> **TIP** For follow-up visits, a nurse or physician's assistant may see you. If your procedure involves a biopsy or other diagnostic test you may receive a follow-up call to let you know the results. Ask your doctor when the results will be available, and if you need to call the office for the results.

What can I do to improve my recovery process (such as changes in my diet, exercising or stopping smoking)?

Where can I get more information about this surgery?

TIP The Surgery Channel web site has information at www.surgerychannel.com, as does WebMD, at www.webmd.com. Just type in the name of the surgery in the search box.

See also: Medication, Pain After Surgery or a Procedure, Pain Questions, and Diagnostic Testing.

Pain After Surgery or a Procedure

Pain is an unpleasant feeling that causes discomfort. Pain serves a purpose; it lets you know that something may be wrong. Without the ability to feel pain, people would be at risk for serious injury. For example, if you did not feel pain, you would not remove your hand from a hot stove.

However, routine pain after a surgery or a procedure is unnecessary, because the cause is known. It is important to have your pain controlled at these times. Good pain control can help you to participate in your own care as you heal. It will also help you to get the proper rest that you will need to heal.

You will play an important part in your pain management. Before surgery, have a discussion with your doctor about pain. Refer to Pain Questions for ideas of how to start the discussion.

Evaluating Pain

No one can know how much pain you are experiencing except you. Your doctor and nurses will be asking you questions about your pain. They may ask you to rate your pain on a scale of 0 to 10. 0 represents the absence of pain, and 10 represents the worst pain you can imagine.

The number that you give will help the doctor and nurses to understand your levels of pain and how the pain medication is helping you.

little pain				increasing pain				most terrible pain	
1	2	3	4	5	6	7	8	9	10

Descriptive words can help your caregivers treat your pain. Words that may be used include burning, stabbing, cramping, pulling, throbbing, pressure, pins and needles.

Be sure to give as much information as possible regarding your pain.

Getting Effective Pain Relief

Patients frequently will refuse pain medication, stating that the pain "isn't that bad yet." They want to hold off and only take the medication when it is absolutely necessary. This is the wrong approach! Pain is very difficult to catch up with; it is much more effective to take pain medication when the pain starts. If you wait until it is too severe, you will require larger doses of medication, and it may be difficult for you to get relief.

Severe pain may make it more difficult for you to participate in your recovery. That could lead to complications that slow your healing.

Complications From Inadequate Pain Control

• Pneumonia can be a complication when you are unable to take deep breaths. After surgery, especially if you had general anesthesia, your breathing is likely to be shallow. This does not allow your lungs to fully expand, and fluid can collect at the base of your lungs. You will likely continue to take shallow breaths if you are in pain. If you have good pain control you will breathe more effectively and may be able to avoid this complication.

• Blood clots sometimes form in patients who are unable to move or to get out of bed for long periods of time. This can be a very dangerous problem, especially if the clot travels to the lung, heart or brain. When your pain is under control you are better able to move, to change positions in bed and to get up out of bed sooner.

• Impaired healing process is a complication from pain. After surgery your body needs to use energy to heal. If your energy is being drained because you are fighting pain, your body has fewer resources to give to the job of healing.

• Skin breakdown and bedsores can be a problem for patients who are not able to get out of bed or to change position in bed. When your pain is managed well, you are more likely to be able to avoid this problem.

Pain Medications

Oral or By Mouth (PO)
This would include pills and liquids that are taken by mouth or are given in a nasogastric tube.

Intravenous (IV)
These medications are given into the patient's IV. IV medications start to relieve pain very quickly after they are given.

Patient-Controlled Analgesia (PCA)
This is IV pain medication that is controlled by the patient. The patient is able to push a button and the pump gives the medication into the IV. The PCA pump ensures that there will not be more medication given than what the doctor ordered. This is one of the most effective ways to control pain in the hospital and can be an excellent method for the first 24 hours after surgery.

Transdermal Patch
This is a patch that contains pain medication. It is applied to your skin and allows small amounts of pain medication to be continuously absorbed through your skin. This is effective for long-term pain control and chronic pain problems.

Intramuscular Injection (IM)
This is commonly known as a "shot." An injection of pain-relieving medication is given with a needle into a muscle, usually in the

buttocks, hip, or arm. This can cause pain at the site of the injection; bleeding and bruising may occur. If you are scheduled to have pain medication regularly, you may prefer to request that the medication be given into your IV.

Side Effects

Powerful medications all have side effects. Unpleasant side effects do not mean that you should stop taking the medication. Your concerns about side effects should be discussed with your doctor before you begin taking the medication. Most side effects can be avoided if you discuss your past medical history with your doctor. If you are having problems with a medication be sure to speak with your doctor or pharmacist.

Please refer to Pain Questions for a list of questions regarding complications or side effects from pain medications.

Addiction

Addiction to narcotics is a very real problem for some people. It is not usually a concern when dealing with acute severe pain from a specific cause. When you are in pain, your body uses narcotics differently than when people take the drugs for recreational purposes. There is very little cause for concern about addiction in these circumstances.

If you have a history of drug or alcohol addiction, discuss this with your doctor. Even with that history, you do not need to be in pain after surgery. Ask for a plan that will meet your needs for pain control.

Overdose

Overdose should not be a concern, as your doctor will be prescribing appropriate doses for you. If you feel confused or overly sleepy while taking your medication, discuss this with your doctor or pharmacist. You may want to ask if the dose that you are taking is usual for someone with your health history. Be sure that the doctor and pharmacist are aware of all the medications and supplements that you are taking. Sometimes medications can interact and cause unexpected side effects. Also, be aware that any amount of alcohol consumed while taking pain medication can increase the risk for overdose.

More information can be found on the Internet. The American Pain Foundation has information on its web site at www.painfoundation.org, as does Hospice.net, at www.hospice.net.

See also: Pain Questions, Medication, Inpatient Surgery, Outpatient Surgery, and Diagnostic Testing.

Pain Questions

What is the pain medication that will be prescribed?

What are the most common side effects of this medication?

How often can I receive pain medication?

Will the medication be given on a schedule, or will I have to ask for it?

> **TIP** Many studies have shown that pain medication is most effective when given on a regular schedule for the first 24 hours after surgery.

Is nausea a side effect of this medication?

What anti-nausea medication will be ordered?

Will the anti-nausea medication be given on a schedule?

> **TIP** Some patients prefer this to prevent nausea rather than to treat it after it has started.

Does the pain medication cause constipation?

Will I be receiving a stool softener or laxative to prevent constipation?

Does this pain medication cause urinary retention?

> **TIP** Some pain medications interfere with the urge to urinate.

What will be done if this pain medication is not effective for me?

How will the pain medication be given?

Pain Medication Can Be Given in Many Ways:

PO
By mouth, this is usually a liquid or pill.

IV
Given into your IV line, the effects are usually felt very quickly.

Transdermal Patch
This is a patch that contains pain medication. It is applied to your skin and allows small amounts of pain medication to be continuously absorbed through your skin.

IM
Intramuscularly; this is a shot (injection) through your skin into a muscle.

> **TIP** If the medication is going to be given more than once, you may want to request that it be given PO or IV, rather than to get several painful injections into your muscle.

Is there a web site or book I can read to get more information on pain control?

> **TIP** The American Pain Foundation has information on its web site at www.painfoundation.org, as does Hospice.net, at www.hospice.net.

See also: Pain After Surgery or a Procedure, Medication, and Getting Along in the Hospital.

Pancreatitis
(Inflammation of the Pancreas)
Questions

What causes pancreatitis?

How is this diagnosis made?

> **TIP** Usually the diagnosis is made with a physical exam, blood tests, urine tests, x-ray, CAT scan, ultrasound or ERCP.

What is an ERCP? Is this necessary to make the diagnosis of pancreatitis?

How can we be sure that I have pancreatitis rather than pancreatic cancer?

What is the treatment for pancreatitis?

What makes me vulnerable to pancreatitis?

Why is it important for me to stop drinking alcohol?

Will pancreatitis make me more likely to develop diabetes or cancer?

Am I likely to have this condition for the rest of my life?

How does my weight affect my condition?

What changes should I make in my diet?

Should I meet with a dietician to help me understand the changes I need to make?

Is it important to stop smoking?

Is there a web site or book I can read to get more information about pancreatitis?

> **TIP** The American Gastroenterological Association has a web site with information at www.gastro.com. WebMD also has information on its web site at www.webmd.com. Just type in *pancreatitis* in the search box.

In the Hospital:

While I am in the hospital, will I need IV fluids?

Do I need to be NPO (nothing by mouth: nothing to eat or drink for a certain period of time)?

> **TIP** Frequently, patients with pancreatitis will be NPO in the hospital because eating can stimulate the pancreas and add to pain.

Will I need to have an NG (nasogastric) tube?

What will I be given for pain control?

Can I have a PCA (patient-controlled analgesia)?

> **TIP** Some experts in the field of pain control recommend PCAs for patients with this type of pain. It can be a very effective way to control the pain while in the hospital.

How long will I be in the hospital?

Will I need surgery?

See also: Pain After Surgery or a Procedure, Pain Questions, Medication, Diagnostic Testing, and Getting Along in the Hospital.

Pediatric Anesthesia

Anesthesia is medication that is given to create a partial or complete loss of sensation or feeling. A licensed anesthesiologist (medical doctor) or certified registered nurse anesthetist administers anesthesia. The following are types of anesthesia:

General
This means that there is a complete loss of sensation and loss of consciousness. The patient cannot feel anything and is unconscious.

General anesthesia requires the placement of a breathing tube and the assistance of a ventilator during surgery. Patients recovering from general anesthesia require monitoring. It is very common to be nauseated after general anesthesia; ask the anesthesiologist what medication may be given to treat nausea.

Your child will not be allowed to eat or drink initially after surgery because general anesthesia causes a temporary decrease in normal bowel function. Depending on the type of surgery your child is to undergo there may be the need to use IV or tube feeding.

Local
Medication given to prevent the feeling of painful sensation in a particular part of the body.

Many people have had a local anesthetic, such as Novocain, from a dentist.

Spinal
Anesthetic medication is given directly into the space around the spinal cord. This blocks pain sensations from below that point on the body.

Epidural

This is similar to a spinal anesthetic. Medication is injected into the space surrounding the spinal cord, temporarily blocking pain from below that point on the body.

The difference between spinal and epidural anesthesia has to do with the space where the medication is injected.

You will meet with your child's anesthesiologist before your child goes to surgery. If possible, arrange to speak with the anesthesiologist several days before your child's surgery so you can have all your questions answered in advance. It is important to know any information about your child's medical history, allergies and how your child has tolerated anesthesia in the past. The anesthesiologist will have you sign a consent form for anesthesia after all your questions have been answered and you understand the process.

More information can be found on the web site Anesthesia Patient Safety at: www.anesthesiapatientsafety.com.

See also: Anesthesia Questions, Pediatric Inpatient Surgery Questions and Pediatric Procedures/Testing Questions.

Pediatric Inpatient Surgery Questions

What is the risk if we do not do the surgery now?

Are there other options for treatment?

> **TIP** You may want to get a second opinion.

What are the risks involved in performing this surgery?

How should I tell my child about this surgery?

> **TIP** Your child's age and level of maturity will affect how and when you discuss the procedure. Ask your pediatrician for advice.

Who will be performing the surgery/procedure?

Will my child need preoperative blood tests? Where can this be done?

What are activity restrictions the day/evening before the procedure?

Does my child need to be NPO (nothing by mouth: nothing to eat or drink for a certain period of time) the evening before the surgery?

Should my child take his regular medications the day of the surgery?

What time should we arrive for the surgery?

How long will we be in the holding room?

TIP You may want to ask if you can be in the holding area where your child will be waiting prior to surgery.

What time will the surgery actually begin?

What are the most common complications related to this procedure?

What is your experience with complications?

What is the mortality rate for this surgery in your hospital?

Does my child's past medical history create risk for complications?

What specific measures are taken to avoid complications?

Will my child need a blood transfusion?

Can family members donate blood for the surgery?

TIP This must be done in advance (usually about a week) and requires a doctor's order.

What type of anesthesia will be used? Are there choices for different types of anesthesia?

Who will be giving the anesthesia?

What types of monitoring devices will be used during this surgery?

How long will the surgery take?

What will happen immediately after the surgery?

Will my child go to the recovery room? How long should I expect him to be in the recovery room?

May I go into the recovery room after my child is awake?

> **TIP** This is a busy place; some hospitals may be reluctant to let you into the recovery room. You may need to be insistent if this is important to you.

How soon after surgery will I be able to see my child?

Should I bring my child's favorite toy to comfort him after the surgery?

Who will keep me informed during the surgery?

> **TIP** Many hospitals have a nurse liaison to keep family members informed during surgery.

What will my child be given to relieve pain after surgery?

What level of pain do patients generally experience immediately after this surgery? The next day? One week later?

Will my child need oxygen or a ventilator after surgery?

What can I expect my child to look like after surgery?

> **TIP** Your child may have monitoring devices and other equipment immediately after surgery.

Will I be able to stay overnight in the hospital with my child?

Will we meet with a discharge planner?

How can I prevent my child from scratching the incision site?

What is the recovery time?

What can I do to improve the recovery process?

How soon can my child return to his normal activities?

Will my child need pain medication while recovering?

Where can I get more information about this surgery?

> **TIP** WebMD has information at www.webmd.com, as does www.anesthesiapatientsafety.com. Just type in the name of the surgery in the search boxes.

See also: Pediatric Procedures/Testing, Pain Questions, Anesthesia, Who's Who in the Healthcare Setting, and Getting Along in the Hospital.

Pediatric Procedures/Testing Questions

Is this test absolutely necessary?

What information will this test give us?

What are the risks involved in performing this procedure or test?

Can I be in the room during the test?

Will my child need an IV?

> **TIP** Some CAT scans and x-rays require IV dye to get better images. You may want to ask your doctor about the possibility of allergic reactions and how this can be avoided.

Do you need to draw blood? Can this be done when the IV is started?

Will my child need to drink anything or take any medication before the test?

Will my child receive sedation before this procedure or test?

Who will give sedation to my child?

Will my child be monitored by a nurse or doctor, and what monitoring devices will be used?

> **TIP** It is especially important that your child's oxygen level be monitored if he receives sedation. Ask if a pulse oximeter will be used to monitor oxygen levels during the procedure.

Should I bring my child's favorite toy or something to comfort him after the procedure?

What is the recovery time after this procedure?

How soon can he return to his normal activities?

What level of discomfort/pain is normal after this procedure?

Will he need medication after the procedure?

Do I need to call to get the results from this test/procedure?

Do you have any additional information that I can read about this type of test?

> **TIP** The Radiological Society of North America has a web site with information about MRI, MRA, CAT scan, x-ray, mammogram and other radiology topics at www.radiologyinfo.org. More information can also be found on WebMD at www.webmd.com. Just type in the name of the test in the search box.

See also: Diagnostic Testing, Pediatric Inpatient Surgery.

Pelvic Inflammatory Disease (PID) Questions

What kind of infection is this?

How did I get it?

What parts of my body are affected?

How serious of an infection is this?

How did you diagnose this? Could it be something else?

How is this treated?

What kind of antibiotics will I take?

Will the antibiotics be in an IV, or will I take them by mouth?

Will I take steroids?

> **TIP** Some doctors recommend steroids to help reduce the painful inflammation. Steroids may also help, in certain cases, to prevent infertility. This may not be true in your specific case.

Will this make me unable to have a baby in the future?

Is this PID a sexually transmitted disease?

Do I need to tell my sexual partner(s) to see a doctor?

If my sexual partner(s) are not treated, will I become reinfected?

How can I prevent having this in the future?

Should I avoid douching?

Is personal hygiene important to prevent the spread of the infection?

What can I do about the pain with this infection?

Will I be given pain medication?

Where can I get more information about PID?

> **TIP** The National Institutes for Health has information on its web site at www.niaid.nih.gov, as does WebMD, at www.webmd.com. Just type in *PID* in the search boxes.

See also: Medication, Pain Questions, and Pain After Surgery or a Procedure.

Peptic Ulcer Disease Questions

What causes peptic ulcer disease?

Do I have the H. pylori infection?

> **TIP** Studies have shown that the majority of patients with peptic ulcers have this infection, which can be treated with antibiotics.

What is the medication that will be prescribed?

How long will I need to take these medications?

What changes to my diet should I begin to make?

> **TIP** Remember to include protein in your diet to help with healthy tissue formation and healing.

Should I lose weight?

Is it important for me to stop smoking?

> **TIP** Smoking can greatly increase the symptoms and severity of peptic ulcer disease.

Should I eliminate alcoholic beverages?

Are there nutritional supplements that I should take?

Is there medication that I should NOT take?

> **TIP** Many doctors advise patients with peptic ulcers to avoid ALL products containing aspirin or ibuprofen (read the labels or ask the pharmacist). You should tell your doctor if you are taking vitamin E or other supplements that may affect your blood clotting.

What are the serious complications that may develop from this condition?

What are the danger signs that I should watch for?

> **TIP** If you experience vomiting of blood, dark, coffee-ground-like vomit, bloody or dark, tarry stools, call your doctor or go to the emergency room—you may have a perforated (or bleeding) ulcer. This can be a life-threatening condition.

Is there information that I can read about peptic ulcers, or a web site where I can obtain more information?

> **TIP** The Centers for Disease Control has information on its web site at www.cdc.gov/ulcer, as does WebMD, at www.webmd.com. Just type in *peptic ulcer* in the search box.

See also: Medication, and Diagnostic Testing.

Peripheral Vascular Disease (PVD) Questions

Why do I have peripheral vascular disease?

> **TIP** Certain people are vulnerable to this; diabetics and renal patients are the two most common groups to develop PVD.

Am I more likely to have problems with sores not healing on my legs and feet?

What precautions should I take to avoid these sores?

> **TIP** Many doctors recommend that people with PVD NEVER wear open-toed shoes and NEVER go barefoot, even in their own homes—because even a small splinter can go unnoticed and develop into a serious infection.

Should I see a podiatrist on a regular basis?

> **TIP** Your doctor may caution you against cutting your toenails or trimming calluses from your feet because of the risk of infection. Many doctors recommend patients with PVD see a podiatrist to care for their feet.

Will insurance and/or Medicare/Medicaid pay for visits to the podiatrist?

What can happen if I develop a sore on my feet that will not heal?

How often should I examine my feet and legs?

> **TIP** If you cannot easily see your feet and the backs of your legs, you may need to ask someone to do this important check for you.

Do you recommend that I lose weight to help this condition?

Are there vitamins and other supplements that could help with this condition?

What type of activities/exercise can I do to help the circulation in my legs and feet?

Does this condition always get worse with time?

How should I alter my eating habits to help my overall health?

> **TIP** Although diet alone cannot cure PVD, frequently patients can experience an increase in health by making small changes to their diets. Be careful to include protein in your diet to help with proper healing and tissue formation.

Are there special shoes or stockings that I should wear?

Will insurance and/or Medicare/Medicaid pay for stockings?

Is this condition likely to become very painful?

What can I do at home to relieve the pain?

Will I be prescribed new medications?

Does having PVD mean that I am more likely to have heart disease or any other serious condition?

Where can I get more information about this condition?

> **TIP** The Society of Cardiovascular and Interventional Radiology has information on its web site at www.sirweb.org. Click on the section for *Patients and the Public* and scroll to *Peripheral Vascular Disease*. WebMD also has information at www.webmd.com. Just type in *PVD* in the search box.

See also: Medication, Pain After Surgery or a Procedure, Pain Questions, and Diagnostic Testing.

Plastic Surgery Questions

Who will be performing the surgery?

> **TIP** As the patient, it is reasonable for you to ask who specifically will be involved in your case.

Is the surgeon board certified in plastic/reconstructive or cosmetic surgery?

How many of these surgeries does the surgeon perform each year?

Should I bring a family member or friend with me on the day of the surgery?

Do I need preoperative blood tests? Where can this be done?

What should I do the day before the surgery?

Do I need to be NPO (nothing by mouth: nothing to eat or drink for a certain period of time) the evening before the procedure?

Should I take my regular medications, including aspirin or vitamins, the day of surgery?

What time should I arrive for the surgery?

Is there a specific place I should park?

What time will the surgery actually begin?

What are the most common complications related to this surgery?

What has been this surgeon's experience with complications?

Does my past medical history create risk for complications?
What specific measures are taken to avoid complications?

What circumstances would make admission to the
hospital necessary?

What type of anesthesia will be used? Do I have options for different
types of anesthesia?

Who will be giving me the anesthesia?

> **TIP** You may ask to speak with the anesthesiologist or nurse anesthetist before
> the day of surgery.

What types of monitoring devices will be used during the surgery?

How long will the surgery take?

What will happen immediately after the surgery?

Will the surgeon check on me in the recovery room to be sure that my
pain is controlled?

How soon after surgery will my family members be able to see me?

When will I be able to go home after the surgery?

What will I be given to relieve pain after surgery?

What level of pain do patients generally experience immediately after
surgery? The next day? One week later?

How much swelling and bruising should I expect after surgery?

Is it possible to have my postoperative prescriptions filled before the surgery?

> **TIP** Be sure you have your pharmacy's phone number with you.

Will I need to arrange transportation home?

Will I need a family member or a friend with me when I return home?

What do I need to know about the recovery process at home?

If I experience problems after I return home, what number should I call?

> **TIP** Problems may include unexpected bleeding, fever or pain not relieved with the pain medication.

When can I start my normal activities, such as exercising, driving and sexual activity?

When can I go back to work?

How many follow-up visits do I need? Will I be seeing the doctor or someone else?

> **TIP** For follow-up visits, a nurse or physician's assistant may see you.

What can I do to improve my recovery process (such as changes in my diet, exercising or stopping smoking)?

Where can I get more information about this surgery?

> **TIP** The Surgery Channel web site has information at www.surgerychannel.com, as does WebMD, at www.webmd.com. Just type in the name of the surgery in the search box.

See also: Medication, Pain After Surgery or a Procedure, Pain Questions, and Outpatient Surgery.

Pneumonia Questions

What is pneumonia?

Is this bacterial or viral pneumonia?

How is that diagnosis made?

> **TIP** Usually, the diagnosis is made after a chest x-ray, sputum culture and blood tests. The doctor will also listen to your lung sounds.

Can you show me on the x-ray what parts of my lungs are affected?

What is my oxygen saturation?

> **TIP** This can be measured by using a pulse oximeter. Typically, healthy individuals have an oxygen saturation of 93% to 100%. With pneumonia, it may be lower because of the infection in your lungs. If it falls below 90%, you may experience confusion and other difficulties due to a lower level of oxygen in your blood.

What treatments/medications will I take to treat the pneumonia?

How long will it take before I feel better?

What complications of pneumonia am I vulnerable to?

How can I avoid these complications?

What should I do if I become more short of breath?

What are the signs that I should call my doctor or go to the emergency room?

Is this contagious?

Are there things about my health or lifestyle that make me vulnerable to pneumonia?

Should I avoid smoking?

Should I avoid secondhand smoke?

Where can I get more information about pneumonia?

> **TIP** The American Lung Association has information on its web site at www.lungsusa.org; click on *Diseases A-Z*. WebMD has information at www.webmd.com. Just type in *pneumonia* in the search box.

See also: Medication, Getting Along in the Hospital, Emergency Room Article, and Emergency Room Visit Questions.

Prostate Disease or
Benign Prostatic Hypertrophy (BPH)

In men, the prostate is a small, walnut-sized organ located below the bladder and in front of the rectum, surrounding the urethra. The urethra is a tube that carries urine from the bladder through the penis and out of the body. The prostate is responsible for the production of fluid for semen, which transports sperm during orgasm.

Symptoms of prostate disease include: the need to urinate frequently, especially at night; difficulty starting urination or holding back urine; inability to urinate; weak or interrupted flow of urine; painful or burning urination; difficulty in having an erection; painful ejaculation; blood in urine or semen; frequent pain or stiffness in the lower back, hips or upper thighs. Any of these symptoms may be caused by cancer or by other, less serious health problems, such as benign prostatic hypertrophy (BPH) or an infection. Early prostate cancer often does not cause symptoms.

Your doctor can screen for prostate disease by performing digital rectal examination and the prostate-specific antigen (PSA) blood test. The American Cancer Society recommends prostate cancer screening for all men over 50 years old and men over 40 who are at high risk, which includes those with a history of prostate cancer in their families.

Up to 65% of men over the age of 64 have BPH. BPH is the abnormal growth of benign (noncancerous) prostate cells. In benign prostatic hypertrophy the prostate grows larger and presses against the urethra and bladder, interfering with the normal flow of urine. BPH is a noncancerous enlargement of the prostate gland that can cause the following symptoms: urinary retention, urinary frequency, dribbling of urine after the stream of urine has stopped, and hesitancy when attempting to urinate. BPH can cause a false-positive result of the PSA test. Other factors such as bacterial infection or prostatitis (inflammation of the prostate) can cause elevated PSA levels, and these must be ruled out in making the diagnosis of prostate disease. It is important to note that a diagnosis of BPH does not necessarily mean that you will have prostate cancer in the future. However, it is important that you continue to be tested for prostate cancer even while being treated for BPH.

Treatment of BPH is with medication or surgery. If symptoms are severe enough, surgical treatment of BPH is considered. The surgical procedure is called transurethral resection of the prostate (TURP) and involves removing tissue from the prostate by inserting an instrument through the urethra into the penis and cutting away the enlarged portions of the prostate. A TURP is performed under general anesthesia and a urine catheter is placed into the penis to empty the bladder. Ask your doctor how the medication or surgery will affect sexual function.

There are many books that can provide more information. There are also several web sites that have helpful information: WebMD has information on its web site at www.webmd.com. Just type *prostate disease* in the search box. More information about prostate cancer can be found on the National Cancer Institute web site at www.nci.nih.gov, as well as on the American Foundation for Urologic Diseases web site at www.afud.org.

See also: Medication, Getting Along in the Hospital, Inpatient Surgery, Depression, Cancer, Diagnostic Testing, and Pain Questions.

Scarlet Fever Questions

What causes scarlet fever?

Is it contagious?

Is this a danger to pregnant women and other adults?

> **TIP** Most adults have developed immunity to the bacteria that causes scarlet fever.

What are the classic symptoms?

What medication will be prescribed?

How long will it take to see improvement in my child's symptoms?

What complications can arise as a result of scarlet fever?

What symptoms should I be watching for in my child?

How should I treat the fever?

How much liquid should my child be drinking with a fever?

> **TIP** Any time your child has a fever, she may become dehydrated if not drinking enough fluids. Signs of dehydration include dry mouth, tearless crying, reduced urination and headache.

Should I be concerned if my child does not want to eat?

Where can I get more information about scarlet fever?

> **TIP** WebMD has information on its web site at www.webmd.com. Just type in *scarlet fever* in the search box. The E-Medicine web site also has information at www.emedicine.com.

See also: Fever in Children, Medication, and Diagnostic Testing.

Seizures Questions

What causes seizures?

> **TIP** Seizures can be caused by problems with the electrical activity in the brain, imbalances in blood chemistry, drug abuse, medication interactions and fevers.

What are the different types of seizures and how are they diagnosed?

> **TIP** You may have a test called an EEG; it measures brain wave activity. Your doctor may also order a CAT scan or an MRI.

What should I tell my friends and family about my seizures?

> **TIP** It is important that you be kept safe while having a seizure. During a seizure you will lose control of all or part of your body; someone should make sure that you do not fall or hit your head.

When is it necessary to call for emergency medical assistance (911)?

Do I need to be brought to the emergency room every time I have a seizure?

Is it important to know how long the seizure lasts?

What is an aura?

What is postictal?

Will I lose control of my bladder and bowels during a seizure?

Will I remember having had a seizure?

Do I need to change my daily activities because of having seizures?

TIP Ask your doctor if you should restrict your driving.

If my child has a history of seizures, should my child's school nurse and/or teachers be aware of it?

Will I need to take medication to prevent seizures?

What are my options for medications?

How will my seizure medications affect the medications I am currently taking?

Should I see a neurologist?

Should I wear a medical alert bracelet?

Am I more likely to have a seizure if I am ill?

Where can I learn more about seizures?

TIP WebMD has information on its web site at www.webmd.com. Just type in the word *seizure* in the search box.

See also: Diagnostic Testing, Emergency Room Visit Questions, Emergency Room Article, and Medication.

Sexually Transmitted Diseases (STD) Questions

These are bacterial, viral, and fungal diseases that are transmitted through sexual contact.

How did I get this disease?

How is the diagnosis made?

> **TIP** Chlamydia, which is one of the most frequently reported infectious diseases, should be diagnosed with either a urine test or a culture; other tests can give false results. Ask you doctor how accurate the testing method is that he uses.

What are the treatments for this disease?

Can I be sexually active while receiving treatment?

Does this treatment cure the disease?

Should I tell my sexual partner(s) that I am being treated for this disease?

What happens if I receive treatment and my partner does not?

> **TIP** Reinfection is likely from sexual contact with an untreated partner.

Do my partners need to be treated if they do not have symptoms?

What happens if I am not treated for this disease?

> **TIP** Women who go untreated for sexually transmitted diseases risk permanent damage to their fallopian tubes and possible sterility. Men and women with untreated syphilis may develop brain damage.

Can birth control prevent STDs?

TIP Proper use of condoms can greatly reduce but not completely eliminate the risk of most STDs.

Will this affect my health in the future?

Will my parents be told I am being treated for an STD?

Where can I get more information about STD's?

TIP WebMD has information on its web site at www.webmd.com. Just type in *sexually transmitted disease*, or the name of the specific disease, in the search box.

See also: Medication Questions and Diagnostic Testing Questions.

Terminology

Anemia

A condition that refers to low hemoglobin in the blood. Hemoglobin carries oxygen in the blood. Anemia can cause fatigue and other symptoms. It can have several causes, such as bleeding or illness.

Anesthesia

Medication that is given to create a partial or complete loss of sensation (feeling). The following are types of anesthesia:

General

This means that there is a complete loss of sensation and loss of consciousness. The patient cannot feel anything and is also unconscious.

General anesthesia usually requires patient consent. General anesthesia requires the placement of a breathing tube and assistance of a ventilator. Patients recovering from general anesthesia require monitoring and special nutrition. It is very common to be nauseated after general anesthesia; you should ask your anesthesiologist what medication you may receive to treat nausea.

> **TIP** You may not be allowed to eat or drink initially after surgery because general anesthesia causes a temporary decrease in normal bowel function.

Local

Medication that is injected into or applied directly on a part of the body to numb it, therefore preventing the sensation of pain.

> **TIP** Many people have had a local anesthetic, such as Novocain, from a dentist.

Spinal

Anesthetic medication is given directly into the space around the spinal cord. This blocks pain sensations from below that point on the body.

Epidural

This is similar to a spinal anesthetic. Medication is injected into the space surrounding the spinal cord, temporarily blocking pain from below that point on the body.

> **TIP** The difference between spinal and epidural anesthesia has to do with the space where the medication is injected.

Antibiotics

Antibiotics are drugs that kill bacteria or stop bacteria from growing.

Arrhythmia

An abnormal rate or rhythm of the heart. It can be felt by some people and is described as a butterfly feeling in the chest. Doctors and nurses use an EKG to determine if someone is having an arrhythmia. Some arrhythmias require monitoring and treatment, and some types do not. It is up to your doctor to determine proper treatment.

Arterial blood gas test (ABG)

This blood test measures precisely how much oxygen is in the patient's blood. It also gives the doctor information about what changes need to be made on the ventilator or in the level of oxygen the patient is receiving.

Artery

A large blood vessel that usually carries blood high in oxygen from the heart to all areas of the body. Arteries have thicker, stronger and more elastic walls than veins.

Arthroscopy

A surgical technique performed by a doctor. An instrument is inserted into a joint to inspect and repair tissue. An arthroscopy is performed on joints, such as knees and shoulders.

Biopsy
During a biopsy a small sample of tissues is taken to be analyzed. This is most frequently done when cancer is a possible diagnosis. Preliminary results from a biopsy may be available immediately after surgery, final results may take a few days.

Blood Transfusion
Blood given to replace blood that has been lost in surgery or due to another cause. Blood is administered in the form of red blood cells or other products such as platelets, or plasma, which help in the clotting process. Patient consent is usually required for blood products to be given, except in the case of emergency.

CAT Scan (Computer Axial Tomography)
This is a series of x-rays taken by a special scanner. The images are computer-analyzed and provide images of the body's organs and structures. The CAT scan provides images from many different angles that a standard x-ray cannot provide.

Chest Tube
A tube approximately the circumference of your little finger. This is inserted into an incision made in the chest wall, usually at the side of the chest. The tube is stitched into place and a thick dressing is applied to the site. The tube allows blood, fluid and air to drain into a collecting chamber.

Complete Bed Rest
A doctor's order that means a patient cannot get out of bed, even to use the bathroom.

Complications
These are difficulties that arise as a result of a surgery, procedure, or just being in the hospital. These can include infection, bleeding, muscle loss due to time spent in bed, as well as many other problems. It is best to ask your doctor or nurse what the most common complications are for your particular case.

Crash Cart

Emergency resuscitation equipment. The crash cart is used during a cardiac arrest and usually includes a defibrillator, emergency drugs and equipment to place an artificial airway (breathing tube).

Discharge Planner

Frequently a nurse or social worker who works with the patient and family to make the appropriate arrangements for the patient's needs after discharge from the hospital. The patient and family may have to ask to see this person. You may ask the discharge planner for assistance in getting in touch with home healthcare agencies and nursing homes, as well as other services.

EKG (Electrocardiogram)

This is a tracing that shows the electrical activity in the heart. It can detect problems such as a heart attack or an irregularity that can lead to an arrhythmia. Small stickers, called leads, are placed on the chest and connected to the EKG machine, which records the electrical activity in the heart.

Heart Monitor (Cardiac Monitor)

Three to five stickers, called leads, are placed on the chest and connected to the heart monitor. This provides a continuous tracing of the electrical activity in the heart, like a continuous EKG. The heart monitor is usually at the bedside and at the nurse's station. The heart monitor allows the doctors and nurses to monitor the rate and rhythm of your heart. Usually alarms will ring if there is something that requires the attention of the doctor or nurse.

Intubation

The placement of a breathing tube and connection to a ventilator.

IV Catheter (Intravenous)

This is a small tube (catheter) that is inserted into your vein. The IV allows fluid and medications to be given directly into your bloodstream. The IV catheter may be in small peripheral veins or in large veins. Usually the nurse will start a new IV every three days to prevent infection.

IV Fluid (Intravenous fluid)
IV fluid is a solution given to provide hydration; it keeps you from being dehydrated. The IV fluid is not usually providing nutrition. Sometimes the fluid has added sugars or salts, but it may be necessary for you to receive nutrition in another manner to help in your healing.

Living Will
A living will is a document that states what medical care and treatments you want and do not want if you are unable to speak for yourself. Every individual has the right to refuse or accept any medical care. The living will allows you to state if you want tube feedings, IV fluids or medications to support your blood pressure. Living will forms can be found on the Internet, at your hospital or from an attorney. See Advance Directives/End-of-Life Decisions.

Nasogastric Tube (NG)
A nasogastric tube is placed into the nose and ends in the stomach. Usually the nasogastric tube is placed on a small amount of wall suction to drain the contents of the stomach. A nasogastric tube may also be used to provide short-term feedings.

MRI (Magnetic Resonance Imaging)
This can provide more detailed information than a standard x-ray image. An MRI uses a large magnet and radio waves to generate an image of internal body structures and organs, especially soft tissues.

Monitoring Devices
This can include any number of devices that monitor bodily functions, such as a heart monitor, automatic blood pressure devices and pulse oximetry.

Pacemaker

This is a device that helps to stabilize the rate that your heart beats. If your heart beats too fast or too slow, a pacemaker can be implanted (internal pacemaker) in your chest to help ensure that your heart rate remains within a safe range. A pacemaker can also be external. External pacing is a temporary measure for patients who need it for a short amount of time, or for patients who are waiting to have an internal pacemaker implanted.

Pulse Oximetry

The pulse oximeter (pulse ox) is a clip that is put on the patient's finger and attaches to a monitor. It gives a constant reading of the level of oxygen in the patient's blood. This does not hurt the patient and can be a good way to monitor the oxygen on a moment-to-moment basis. Variation in oxygen levels let the healthcare professionals know that changes in the ventilator or oxygen delivery may be needed. Ideally, the pulse ox reading is 90 to 100%, but some patients live with lower readings. Each patient is an individual case.

Suctioning

If a breathing tube is inserted, it may be necessary for the doctor, nurse or respiratory therapist to suction the patient. A smaller tube is passed down the breathing tube, and gentle suction is applied. This helps to clear the patient's airway of fluid or secretions. This is necessary because patients who are on a ventilator can have difficulty coughing and clearing their throat of fluid secretions. Different catheters can be used to suction the mouth or nose.

Surgical Holding Room

An area near the operating room where patients are brought prior to surgery. The holding area is the place where the IV will be started and where other procedures may be done prior to going to the operating room.

Urine Catheter

This is frequently referred to as a "Foley" catheter. The tube is inserted into the bladder to drain urine. The urine drains from the tube into an attached bag. The bag is usually hung on the side of the hospital bed. Frequently, the tube is taped to the patient's leg to help it stay in place. A urinary catheter should not prevent the patient from getting up, walking or sitting in a chair, if he is not on complete bed rest.

Ventilator

The ventilator is a machine that either completely or partially assists the patient in breathing. See Ventilator Information.

Vital signs

Vital signs are your heart rate, respiratory rate (breathing), blood pressure and temperature. Some hospitals consider pain levels to be the fifth vital sign.

Vitamins

Supplements that are usually taken without a prescription to provide important substances that are essential for proper metabolism, growth and development. Some vitamins and minerals and other nutritional supplements, such as vitamins E and C
and other antioxidants, affect how the blood clots. This can be
very beneficial for some people, but it can have an impact on recovery
from surgery. Please discuss all of the supplements that
you are taking with your doctor before surgery. Other supplements, such as St. John's Wort, interact with prescription drugs; your doctor should be aware of what you are taking, so as to avoid possible problems.

X-rays

These are radiographic images of specific body parts. X-rays are useful for viewing solid body structures, such as bones. They can also be used to view lungs and other organs.

Tonsillectomy Questions

What is the function of the tonsils and adenoids? Will they both be removed?

Do tonsils and adenoids grow back after surgery?

Why is this procedure necessary?

Is there an alternative to surgery?

What is the risk if I don't have surgery?

What are the risks involved with having this surgery?

What are the most common complications with tonsillectomies?

How long will the procedure take?

Will I have the surgery if I have a cold?

Is general anesthesia necessary?

Will I go home the day of the procedure?

What problems should I watch for after surgery?

How much blood is expected or normal to be spitting out the day after surgery?

> **TIP** When blood mixes with saliva, it can look like there is a lot of bleeding. Ask your doctor how much is to be expected.

165

What should I do if I experience nausea and vomiting at home after surgery?

> **TIP** Children may swallow blood and become nauseated. Ask your doctor what the signs are of excessive blood loss in children.

Should I call the doctor's office if I develop a fever after surgery?

> **TIP** Typically, a doctor will want to be notified if your temperature is greater than 101.5 after surgery. Ask your doctor what is the best method to take your temperature.

Should someone be with me for the first 24 hours after surgery?

How much pain is to be expected after surgery?

What medications will I be taking after surgery?

Where can I get more information about tonsillectomy?

> **TIP** WebMD has information on its web site at www.webmd.com. Just type in *tonsillectomy* in the search box.

See also: Outpatient Surgery, Medication, Pain After Surgery or a Procedure, Pain Questions, Pediatric Procedures/Testing, and Pediatric Anesthesia.

Transplant Surgery Questions

The following questions are general and are meant to help you to start a conversation with your doctor about transplant surgery. They may not all apply to your specific circumstances; choose the questions that are helpful for you.

What are the alternatives to surgery?

How will my past medical history affect the surgical outcome?

What medications will I need to take before the transplant?

What medications will I need to take after the transplant?

Will I be on these medications for the rest of my life?

What side effects will I have from taking these medications?

What is the cost of these medications?

Does insurance or Medicare/Medicaid pay for these medications? (If so, for how long will they cover the cost?)

How often will I need blood tests before/after surgery?

How often will I need to see the doctor before/after surgery?

Are there foods, medication, over-the-counter drugs or alcoholic beverages I should avoid?

How long will I be in surgery?

How long will I be in the hospital?

Will I need physical rehabilitation after surgery?

Are there specific things I can do to keep myself healthy before the surgery?

> **TIP** Ask your doctor about seeing a dietician before surgery. It is beneficial to have good nutritional habits prior to a major surgery.

What changes in my lifestyle will I have after surgery?

Tell me about the surgical procedure and the postoperative course.

Will I need a blood transfusion?

Can my family or I give a directed blood donation before surgery?

> **TIP** This will need to be done with a written order from your doctor; planning on this should be weeks ahead of the surgery.

Are there support groups for transplant patients that my family and I can attend?

Can you help me to meet someone that has had this transplant so I can hear first hand what my life will be like after the transplant?

Where can I get more information about this surgery?

> **TIP** The National Transplant Assistance Fund has information on its web site at www.transplantfund.org, as does WebMD, at www.webmd.com. Just type in the name of the surgery in the search box.

See also: Inpatient Surgery, Getting Along in the Hospital, Pain After Surgery or a Procedure, Pain Questions, and Anesthesia.

Urinary Tract Infection (UTI), Bladder Infection/Cystitis in Children and Adults Questions

What causes a UTI?

What are the symptoms of a UTI?

How is the diagnosis made?

> **TIP** Usually the doctor will need a "midstream clean-catch" urine sample. Women will be asked to clean themselves wiping from front to back with a special pad, then urinate in the toilet, and then urinate in the sterile cup provided to you. It is important that you are clean and that you catch your urine midstream.

What is the treatment for a UTI?

Will I need an IV?

What medication can I take to treat the discomfort I feel?

Does this affect just my lower urinary tract?

> **TIP** Some urinary tract infections can spread and affect the upper urinary tract and kidneys. This can be a serious illness and requires different treatment than a simple UTI.

Should I watch for fever, vaginal discharge, back pain and/or blood in the urine?

How much water should I drink every day to avoid another UTI?

Will increasing the amount of protein and fruits that I eat help to prevent a UTI?

> **TIP** Protein and fruits increase a beneficial acid in your urine that can help to prevent UTI.

Should I avoid beverages with high sugar content, such as soda and juices?

Is it important to avoid bubble baths?

For women: Should I urinate after sexual intercourse to avoid UTI?

For men: Can a UTI indicate there is a problem with my prostate?

What other information can you give me about urinary tract infections?

> **TIP** The American Academy of Pediatrics has a web site with more information at www.aap.org. There is also more information on the National Institutes of Health web site at www.niddk.nih.gov. Just type in *urinary tract infection* in the search boxes.

Ventilator Information

What is it?

The ventilator is a machine that either completely or partially assists the patient in breathing. Oxygen is supplied through a tube that is attached to the ventilator and inserted down the patient's throat. This is usually a temporary way of helping the patient breathe. The tube brings oxygen to the patient's lungs (inhalation) and removes carbon dioxide from them (exhalation). The tube also allows the healthcare professionals (doctors, nurses and respiratory therapists) to suction the patient's airway to keep it clear of fluid and secretions. Ventilators are used often in surgery because anesthetic agents may make it impossible for the patient to breathe without assistance.

What does it do?

The ventilator can either assist the patient's breathing (in cases where the patient is unable to effectively breathe), or it may be doing all of the work of breathing for the patient. Sometimes patients are too sick to protect their airway; they might choke if left to breathe on their own. In that case the patient would be intubated, i.e., the breathing tube would be put down the patient's throat, and the ventilator would be attached, providing extra oxygen and giving the patient a breath when needed, but the patient would be starting most of his breaths. The ventilator would just be a safety precaution until the patient is strong enough to breathe entirely alone.

Sometimes patients are extremely ill and need to have all of the work of breathing done by the ventilator. These patients usually are sedated with medications that help them rest and stay calm. Patients who are extremely ill need to use all of their energy toward healing. The ventilator can help the patient use his energy for getting well rather than for breathing.

Complications

Patients who are using a ventilator are usually very sick or have a serious injury. Patients in this condition are more sensitive to infections such as pneumonia. This can be treated with antibiotics, but it is an extra stress on sick patients.

Being on a ventilator can also increase the pressure in the lungs. This can lead to a condition called pneumothorax, or collapsed lung. There are very effective treatments for this condition. The most common treatment is inserting a chest tube, which releases some of the pressure and allows the collapsed lung to reinflate.

Patients on a ventilator are usually receiving more benefit from the ventilator than problems. Most patients who are on ventilators for short periods of time do not experience these problems.

Measuring Progress

There are tests and procedures that the ventilated patient will have, usually every day, sometimes more frequently.

• Chest X-ray—usually done every day. This allows the healthcare professionals to view the patient's lungs. It shows that the tube is in the proper place and whether there is a buildup of fluid in the lungs. The chest x-ray helps the doctor know if the lungs are damaged or getting healthier.

• Blood Tests—an arterial blood gas (ABG) test may be drawn every day or every few hours, if necessary. This blood test measures precisely how much oxygen is in the patient's blood. It also gives the doctor information about what changes need to be made on the ventilator.

• Pulse Oximetry—the pulse ox is a clip that is put on the patient's finger and attaches to a monitor. It can give a constant reading of the level of oxygen in the patient's blood. This does not hurt the patient and can be a good way to monitor the oxygen on a moment-to-moment basis. Changes in this number let the healthcare professionals know that changes in the ventilator may be needed. Ideally, the pulse ox reading is 90 to 100%, but some patients live with lower readings. Each patient is an individual case.

• Suctioning—it will be necessary for the doctor, nurse or respiratory therapist to suction the patient. A smaller tube is passed down the breathing tube, and gentle suction is applied. This helps clear the patient's airway of fluid or secretions. This is necessary because a patient who is on a ventilator can have difficulty coughing and clearing his throat of secretions or fluid.

More information can be found on the WebMD web site at www.webmd.com. Just type in the word *ventilator* in the search box.

See also: Ventilator Questions, Pain Questions, and Advance Directives/End-of-Life Decisions.

Ventilator Questions

The ventilator is a machine that either completely or partially assists the patient in breathing. Oxygen is supplied through a tube that is attached to the ventilator and inserted down the patient's throat. This is usually a temporary way of helping the patient breathe. The tube brings oxygen to the patient's lungs (inhalation) and removes carbon dioxide from them (exhalation). The tube also allows the healthcare professionals (doctors, nurses and respiratory therapists) to suction the patient's airway to keep it clear of fluid and secretions. Ventilators are used often in surgery because anesthetic agents may make it impossible for the patient to breathe without assistance.

Why is the ventilator necessary?

How long do you think that the ventilator will be needed?

How much oxygen is being given?

How much support is the ventilator providing? Is it partial or complete support?

What are the complications that could develop because of the ventilator?

What is being done to avoid these complications?

How often should the patient be suctioned?

How is the need for nutrition being met?

TIP This is an important question; the IV fluids are not nutrition.

Are there complications from this type of nutritional support?

Is a dietician being consulted?

Will the patient need additional sedation while on the ventilator?

How do you know if the patient is in pain?

Will the patient need to have his hands restrained while on
the ventilator?

> **TIP** This is a common safety practice to prevent the patient from removing the breathing tube.

Will the patient be able to get out of bed while on the ventilator?

What can be done to help the patient get off the ventilator?

Who will decide when it is safe to take the patient off
the ventilator?

Is there a web site or book where I can get more information
about ventilators?

> **TIP** More information can be found on the WebMD web site at www.webmd.com. Just type in *ventilator* in the search box.

See also: Advance Directives/End-of-Life Decisions, Pain Questions,
Ventilator Information, Getting Along in the Hospital, and
Nutritional Support.

What's in the Chart

The illness and hospitalization of a loved one can be a scary and confusing time. It can be tempting to think that mysteries will be solved if you could just get a look at the chart. Usually the chart will not provide a good deal of information to people who are not medically trained. Your best chance for coherent information is to have a written list of questions that you would like to ask the doctor and nurses.

The following is a general listing of what is contained in most medical charts. With the advent of computerized charting, this may not exist in paper form.

Physician's Orders
These pages contain specific orders for the patient's medications and other treatments.

Progress Notes
These pages are used by all healthcare professionals to keep a narrative record of the patient's progress or unusual events. Generally they contain medical terminology and abbreviations, most of which is usually not understood by non-medically trained people. A better understanding of the patient's condition can be obtained by speaking with a doctor or nurse.

Laboratory Results
Usually a computer-generated record of all of the laboratory results for the patient's entire hospital stay.

Consents

Documents that are signed by the patient giving healthcare professionals permission to perform certain tests or procedures. A consent may be needed before surgery or an invasive procedure such as a biopsy. Signing a consent means the procedure has been fully explained and that the risks and benefits of treatment are understood. If the patient is unable to sign or incapable of signing, consent is given by the spouse or next of kin. Not all procedures require a consent form. If you are concerned about any type of procedure—please ASK!

Miscellaneous

Most charts will contain various other sections such as surgical records. Surgery records contain information about vital signs, drugs administered, IVs and catheters that were placed during surgery.

What to Ask at
Your Next Doctor's Appointment

Everyone has individual concerns prior to going to the doctor. Here are some questions to help you to start a conversation about your long-term health. Be sure to bring a list of questions to ask your doctor with you to the appointment, and jot down the doctor's answers. It can be difficult to remember your questions and the doctor's answers if they are not written down.

Do I have risk factors for developing serious health problems?

> **TIP** Your habits, family history and past medical problems may make it more likely that you will develop certain medical conditions. You may be able to prevent these conditions if you adjust your lifestyle or make other changes.

Am I at risk for Type 2 diabetes?

> **TIP** Type 2 diabetes is at an epidemic level in the United States. There are ways to prevent it; ask your doctor for more information.

Do you recommend that I lose weight? What is the best way to lose weight?

Can I participate in an exercise program? What do you suggest?

How often should I have blood tests done? Should I have my cholesterol levels checked?

> **TIP** Some other blood tests that you may want to ask about are:
> - Complete Blood Count (CBC)
> - Cholesterol
> - Blood Glucose (blood sugar)
> - Electrolytes
> - PSA (blood test for indications of prostate cancer)
> - CA125 (blood test for indications of ovarian cancer)

Should I have an EKG, mammogram, chest x-ray, colonoscopy or any other diagnostic tests?

Should I have my stool tested for hidden blood?

> **TIP** This is a very quick, painless and important test to help screen for colon cancer. This is called the hemocult stool test.

May I have copies of all of my test results?

> **TIP** This can be especially helpful for patients who have changes in doctors and insurance carriers every few years. If you keep track of the important test results, you will have more control over your long-term health history.

Is it necessary to have a yearly checkup even if I feel well?

Is it necessary to have a formal yearly checkup even if I have seen the doctor when I was ill during the year?

> **TIP** Generally, seeing the doctor because of cold or flu symptoms does not take the place of the formal yearly checkup. When you see the doctor for illness, he is not necessarily focused on your overall health outlook, and important tests may not be performed.

Should I continue taking all of the medications that I currently take?

> **TIP** Be sure to bring a list of all the medications that you are taking, including vitamins, supplements, and over-the-counter medications. It is important that your doctor is aware of everything that you are taking. Keep a list of all your current medications in your wallet at all times.

Do you recommend that I get any immunizations?

> **TIP** Your doctor may recommend that you receive a flu shot every year in the fall months. You may also ask about the hepatitis B vaccine; it is recommended for people who may be at a greater risk of contracting hepatitis B because of lifestyle or job description.

Do you recommend that I occasionally have my blood pressure checked?

> **TIP** This can be easily done in many communities at local pharmacies or in shopping malls. Ask your doctor if you should keep a record of blood pressure readings that are done in between doctor's appointments.

Do you have any other recommendations that will benefit my long-term health?

Would you describe me as being in good health?

See also: Medication, and Diagnostic Tests.

When Someone You Love
Is in the Hospital

There are many reasons why you or a loved one may be hospitalized. The following questions are general and are meant to help you start a conversation with the doctor in the hospital. They may not all apply to your loved one's specific circumstances; choose the questions that are helpful for you. For simplicity, we have referred to the patient as "he" in these questions.

How long will he be in the hospital?

What tests are being done?

Can we have a copy of blood tests, x-rays, and CAT scans?

> **TIP** It is a good idea to get copies of tests to keep with your loved one's medical records. This is also helpful so that you can compare the test results to results of previous tests. It is usually not a problem to get blood test results in the hospital; they are easily printed out of the computer. The patient will need to give his permission for you to obtain copies of the tests unless you are the medical power of attorney (see Advance Directives/End-of-Life Decisions). Copies of x-rays and CAT scans may require a formal written request.

What other doctors are involved in his care?

> **TIP** The patient may be seen by other specialists while in the hospital; you may ask to meet with them.

Is there evidence of an infection?

> **TIP** Older patients who are suddenly confused or lethargic may have an infection; this may be pneumonia or a urinary tract infection.

How will the infection be treated?

Will he be allowed to eat?

How will his nutrition needs be met?

> **TIP** People who are ill have an increased need for nutrition. IV fluid is not nutrition.

Will he be seen by a physical therapist?

> **TIP** Even a couple of days of bed rest can severely weaken muscles, especially in older patients. It is reasonable to ask if physical therapy will be included in the treatment.

Will there be a need for rehabilitation after discharge from the hospital?

Will there be a change in his medications while he is in the hospital?

Will he need to continue new medications at home?

Will he need to make changes in his diet at home?

Will he see a dietician while in the hospital?

Should we see a discharge planner or a social worker to plan for discharge?

What plans need to be made to take the patient home?

> **TIP** If you will need special equipment or help at home caring for the patient, it is best to start planning for that early in the hospitalization.

See also: Diagnostic Testing, Medication, Pain Questions, Discharge Planning, and Advance Directives/End-of-Life Decisions.

Who's Who in the Healthcare Setting

Anesthesiologist
A physician who has received advanced training in the delivery of anesthesia. The anesthesiologist monitors patients under anesthesia for subtle changes in oxygen levels or cardiac status.

TIP Not all anesthesia needs to be administered by an anesthesiologist.

Attending Physician (MD)
An attending physician is a practicing doctor who has seniority in a teaching hospital and has privileges to admit patients to a particular hospital. The attending physician may also hold board certifications in various areas of specialty, indicating advanced training in those areas.

Dietician
A person specifically trained and licensed in the science of nutrition and health. Dieticians can be a valuable resource in the hospital for physicians and patients to call upon for detailed nutrition information and resources. Dieticians are especially good resources to consult for managing chronic illness from a nutrition standpoint.

Fellow (MD)
In a teaching hospital, or a hospital affiliated with one, fellows are doctors in training. A fellow is a physician that has completed residency training; fellowships are advanced training programs that provide an intensive focus on a specific area of medicine, such as cardiology or transplantation. Fellowship programs vary in length, depending on the specialty. Frequently the fellow will supervise a group of residents in a teaching hospital.

Intern (MD)

A first-year graduate from medical school. An intern, who functions with supervision from residents and attending physicians, may only perform specific duties. An internship lasts one year and progresses to residency.

Nurse Anesthetist

A registered nurse with education and certification in the delivery of anesthesia. Nurse anesthetists work under the direct or indirect supervision of an anesthesiologist.

Patient Care Technician (PCT)

These individuals are unlicensed assistive personnel who are trained by the hospital (or other training programs) to aid in the care of patients. PCTs typically function with the supervision of a registered nurse. Their duties may include measuring temperature, pulse or blood pressure, assisting patients in and out of bed, and walking with patients in the hallway. Institutions may also refer to workers in this role as nursing assistants (NA) or patient care assistants (PCA). Some institutions may use PCTs to do EKGs and blood draws, and to set up oxygen therapy.

Pharmacist

A pharmacist has advanced training and education in the preparation of medications. A pharmacist is an excellent resource for information about the uses, interactions and effects of medications.

Physical and Occupational Therapist (PT and OT)

Physical Therapists and Occupational Therapists are specifically trained and licensed to help patients regain or maintain strength in their muscles and limbs. PTs and OTs have the goal to restore function and prevent disability.

Physician's Assistant (PA)

A physician's assistant is a person trained in specific aspects of medical practice to provide assistance to a physician. Specifically trained (and in some cases licensed), physician's assistants perform tasks that would otherwise need to be performed by an MD. Physician's assistants work in many areas of the healthcare industry.

Radiology Technician

A person trained and licensed to perform x-rays, CAT scans, MRIs, and various other radiological procedures ordered by physicians.

Registered Nurse (RN)

A registered nurse has received education and training for a Bachelor's Degree, Associate Degree or Diploma Program in nursing. Registered nurses must pass state licensure exams. Nurses work in the hospital and in outpatient care settings, providing a variety of care and monitoring functions. Nurses are skilled in many areas and may obtain certification to provide specific care.

Resident (MD)

Residents are physicians who have graduated from medical school, completed an internship and are licensed to practice medicine. Lengths of residency programs vary, depending on the specialty. Residents are assigned to a specific hospital or hospital system in which to practice and are supervised by attending physicians and fellows. Residents are termed house staff in the hospital where they practice.

Respiratory Therapist (RT)

Respiratory therapists are trained to administer medications, oxygen and treatments to improve and maintain pulmonary (lung) function. Respiratory therapists work in a variety of healthcare settings primarily in hospitals. Respiratory therapists are part of the healthcare team and give input and recommendations into a patient's care.

Social Worker

In most states this individual has a Master's Degree and is licensed to practice social work. A social worker functions in many roles in various healthcare settings. In the hospital, a social worker is typically involved in the process of preparing for discharge to home or an extended care facility. In the hospital, social workers may help to manage and oversee patients with specific disease categories. Social workers may arrange for home health visits and for home care equipment. Social workers can be a source of information regarding reimbursement for services from Medicare and insurance. Patients and families are able to request the services of a social worker.

About the Authors

Margaret Fitzpatrick, RN is a trauma nurse specialist with experience in the fields of inpatient hospice care, surgical intensive care, emergency and trauma care and school nursing.

Ms. Fitzpatrick was honored in 2002 by the Chicago City Council for actions related to her work as a school nurse.

Linda Burke, RN is a registered nurse with years of experience in cardiac care and surgical and trauma intensive care as well as in training nurses new to the field of critical care nursing.

Daryl Lee, RN is a registered nurse who has experience working in surgical and trauma intensive care and medical intensive care.